OTOLARYNGOLOGY RESEARCH ADVANCES

HANDBOOK OF HEARING DISORDERS RESEARCH

Otolaryngology Research Advances

Additional books in this series can be found on Nova's website under the Series tab.

Additional e-books in this series can be found on Nova's website under the e-book tab.

OTOLARYNGOLOGY RESEARCH ADVANCES

HANDBOOK OF HEARING DISORDERS RESEARCH

CHARLOTTE HAILEE ATKINSON
EDITOR

Nova Biomedical
New York

NOTICE TO THE READER

Library of Congress Cataloging-in-Publication Data

ISBN: 978-1-63463-654-4

Library of Congress Control Number: 2014956988

Published by Nova Science Publishers, Inc. † New York

Contents

Preface

Deafness is one of the most widespread, costly and poorly understood disabilities in the world. Hearing impairment is a condition that involves medical, psychological and social aspects. According to the World Health Organization (WHO) about 250 million people have disabling hearing loss and two-thirds of them live in the developing world. Millions of people progressively lose their most important means of communication and became socially isolated, especially in the later years of their life. This handbook provides recent research on several different hearing disorders.

Chapter 1 – Research into the effect of hearing loss (HL) on traffic safety and mobility is limited and the empirical findings are somewhat inconsistent. HL is one of the most frequent sensory deficits in humans, leading to loss of auditory information, which may affect behavior in traffic situations and might reduce traffic safety and mobility. The prevalence of age-related HL in Europe is roughly 30% for men and 20% for women at the age of 70 years, and 55% for men and 45% for women at the age of 80 years. The prevalence of age-related HL is increasing, and as a consequence the number of road users with HL will also increase.

The aim of this PhD thesis was to investigate traffic safety and mobility for individuals with HL. Three studies were conducted: 1. a questionnaire survey aimed to evaluate differences in choice of transportation that might be related to HL, 2. a driving simulator study that looked into compensatory strategies and evaluated the efficiency of a tactile signal to alert the driver, and 3. a field study to evaluate these effects in real traffic and to evaluate a navigation system with a supportive tactile signal.

The results of the three studies indicate that there are effects of HL on traffic safety and mobility. The effects are relatively small and often bound to driving complexity; but, systematic and consistent in replicated study. Differences in transportation habits related to HL include less likelihood of having a driver's license and a higher valuing of written information, with the latter possibly prioritized before time and safety issues. Moreover, respondents with more HL were less concerned about the effects of HL, which suggests that they might be using compensatory strategies.

In the experimental studies, differences in driving behavior related to HL were bound to driving conditions and occurred when the complexity of the driving task increased. There was also an effect of HL on visual behavior, indicated in the simulator and confirmed in the field study, suggesting that drivers with HL have more active visual behaviors with more frequent glances in the rear-view mirror and a general scanning of the environment before looking away from the road. A tactile signal in the driver seat was found useful in both experimental studies, both for calling for the driver's attention and facilitating navigation using a GPS navigation device.

It was concluded that there are effects of HL on both traffic safety and mobility, consistently pointing toward a generally more cautious driving behavior with the use of both compensatory and coping strategies, which suggests a difference in experienced safety. Compensatory strategies associated with HL include driving at lower speeds and using a more comprehensive visual search behavior. Coping strategies associated with HL include engaging less in distracting activities. Evaluation of the tactile signal suggests that it may make driver assistance systems more accessible, not only to drivers with HL, but to all drivers. At the same time, the systems might become more effective for all users, since visual resources can be more focused on the road, which could increase both traffic safety and mobility in general.

Chapter 2 – There is a growing awareness that a variety of different chemical substances can cause hearing damage in humans. The literature of the last decade on the effect of different chemical compounds on the human auditory system has been reviewed with reference to the exposure in the workplace. Scientific evidence has emerged that the exposure to styrene, p-xylene, solvent mixtures and lead may be a cause of hearing loss. For these substances the number of studies is relatively large and a variety of approaches have been undertaken to test their effect on the auditory system. For other chemical substances, for example certain metals such as mercury, cadmium and arsenic, and some neurotoxic pesticides, the available data indicate a possible ototoxic action, although in some cases only when in combination with noise. A number of critical aspects have been noticed: firstly, this review highlights the need to consider the possible synergistic effect of the interactions between different ototoxic agents, primarily the co-exposure to noise. These interactions are complex and difficult to predict, since synergistic, additive and sub-additive effects have to be contemplated. Then, the individual variability of exposed subjects, due to genetic differences, personal clinical histories, and occupational/environmental exposures cannot be disregarded. Finally, there are conceptual differences among the studies in the definition of hearing loss, which may partly account for the different prevalence values found in the examined documents. In conclusion, it is suggested to adopt the precautionary principle, while awaiting, on one hand, a stronger evidence on the ototoxicity of some classes of chemicals, particularly for exposures at low doses, and, on the other hand, new scientific studies on the effects of the interaction between physical and chemical agents on the hearing loss that are a priority in future research needs.

Chapter 3 – Sudden sensorineural hearing loss (SSNHL) is an important cause of acquired hearing deficits in the adults. Several pathophysiological hypothesis have been proposed so far, however the cause of sudden hearing loss is still unclear. Even if local hypoxic/ischemic events as well as inner ear viral infection have been reported to be the main hypothesis leading to transient or permanent cochlear dysfunction, and therefore to Sudden Sensorineural Hearing Loss, still there are other hypothesis that have been claimed.

Aim of the present study is to investigate about the possible role of iron metabolism, and in particular about the presence of genetic variants of the principal iron-related genes, and acute inner ear disorders such as sudden sensorineural hearing loss.

Chapter 4 – The cochlea is especially sensitive to circulatory alterations because it is supplied by a single terminal artery and lacks adequate collateral blood supply.

To examine the putative association between Sensorineural Hearing Loss (SNHL) and Sleep Disordered Breathing (SDB) through the literature review is very interesting.

In fact these medical disorders usually are associated to cerebral circulatory alterations resulting in hypoxia, acute hemodynamic change, and decreased cerebral blood flow, because the Sleep Disorder Breathing (SDB), for example OSAHS (Obstructive Sleep Apnea Hypopnea Syndrome), is characterized by periodic hyposia/reoxygenation. These noxious stimuli can, in turn, activate the sympathetic nervous system, depress parasympathetic activity which results in oxidative stress, endothelial dysfunction, and activation of the inflammatory cascade of different anatomical structure as inner ear. Is reasonable to assume that could cause and/or esacerbate sensorineural hearing loss with/or without tinnitus.

Based on these clinical evidences some authors studied the association between SDB and a dysfunction of auditory pathway showing an improved risk of sensorineural hearing loss, a lower transient otoacoustic emissions (TEOAE) reproducibility and an impairment of auditory brainstem responses in OSAHS populatio. In fact it is known that the transduction mechanism of the inner ear and the transmission of nerve impulses along the auditory way are highly dependent upon the oxygen supply. Recent studies evidenced how through oxidative injury due to a hypoxic stress induced apoptosis in spiral ligament and in the cochlear basal turn of the Organ of Corti of obese CD/1 mouses, causes a high frequencies sensorineural hearing loss.

Therefore OSAHS may lead to cerebral vascular insufficiency resulting in hypoxia, acute hemodynamic change, and decreased cerebral blood flow during episodes of apnea with consequent ischemic injury to the cochlea.

Chapter 5 – Tinnitus is a common symptom in individuals of various age groups, but the impact it causes is variable, depending on the characteristics of subjects. The aim of this study is to analyze the characteristics of tinnitus and the discomfort it causes in individuals assessed in a specific outpatient clinic in a tertiary hospital. Participants were evaluated by medical history interview, medical examination, grading of tinnitus severity, hearing screening and testing, measurement of tinnitus pitch and loudness and THI instrument for identifying tinnitus discomfort. The sample consisted of 199 individuals; 124 of them (62.30%) were females, with a mean age of 58.18 ± 12.79 years, with bilateral tinnitus (50.8%) and average length of tinnitus presence was 5.18 ± 4.67 years. Tinnitus pitch was acute and tinnitus loudness was moderate, within the values reported in the technical literature. Mean tinnitus severity was 5.18 ± 4.67 years and the THI score ranged from 0 to 98 points (mean 40.03 ± 25.48 points). No difference was observed between THI scores and sex and tinnitus location. Correlation was observed between tinnitus severity and THI scores, between age and tinnitus loudness in the left ear, and between age and THI scores.

Chapter 6 – Dominant deafness-onychodystrophy syndrome (DDOD, MIM 124480) is a type of ectodermal dysplasia characterized mainly by congenital deafness, absent nails and/or toes with variable presence of brachydactyly, hypoplastic distal phalanges, and bulbous distal phalanges. Using the whole-exome sequencing approach, the authors identified a de novo mutation (c.1516 C>T [p.Arg506X]) in ATP6V1B2 as the cause of DDOD syndrome in three independently identified individuals. Molecular epidemiology analysis showed that the ATP6V1B2 p.Arg506X mutation was not present in 1053 ethnically matched normal hearing controls. ATP6V1B2 encodes a component of the vacuolar ATPase (V-ATPase, also known as H+-ATPase), a multisubunit enzyme that mediates acidification of eukaryotic intracellular organelles. The authors generated an Atp6v1b2 knockdown mouse model and found that

Atp6v1b2 deficiency leads to severe sensorineural hearing loss. In vitro pathogenic evaluation showed that the ATP6V1B2 p.Arg506X mutation is a dominant haplo-insufficient mutation that caused abnormal acidification in the lysosomes. The acidification defect in lysosomes may cause decreased activity of acid-dependent hydrolases and thus hydrolytic dysfunction of the lysosome affects development of multiple systems such as the inner ear, phalanx, and nail in the DDOD syndrome. The findings provide the molecular basis for DDOD genetic diagnosis as well as exciting developments in future therapeutic interventions.

Chapter 7 – Identifying the genetic basis of deafness provides crucial information for diagnosis, intervention and treatment of the disease. Non-syndromic sensorineural hearing loss, however, are extremely heterogeneous, with both common and rare forms occurring due to mutations over estimated 500 genes. Due to the larger number and presumably low mutation frequencies of those genes, it would be highly expensive and time-consuming to address this issue by conventional gene-by-gene Sanger sequencing. Next generation sequencing (NGS) has become a highly efficient strategy for identifying novel causative genes and mutations involved in heritable disease. Both simple nonsyndromic and complex syndromic forms of hearing loss can be resolved efficiently using NGS, especially in small families with distinct and interesting phenotypes that were once too small to map. To date, more than a dozen syndromic or nonsyndromic deafness genes have been identified using targeted genomic enrichment and NGS. Here, the authors summarized novel deafness genes and mutations identified by NGS methodologies.

Chapter 8 – Hearing impairment is a condition that involves medical, psychological and social aspects. Surveys report that children and adolescents with hearing impairment show high prevalence of psychopathology. Among numerous definitions which are largely overlapping (Oppositional Defiant Disorders, Externalizing Disorder, Behavior Problems, Socio-emotional Problems), the authors have chosen the definition of conduct disorder given by the World Health Organization in ICD -10. Some of the criteria for the diagnosis are: violation of the rules of adults, frequent anger and resentment, deliberate destruction of other people's property. The aim of this paper is to examine the relationships between hearing impairment and conduct disorder. The survey was conducted in Serbia, the environment characterized by specific circumstances concerning the educational and socio-economic conditions. This society has not developed a tradition of inclusive education for children, and inclusive trends are slow in general. The study was conducted on 375 patients of whom 169 are with a hearing impairment, and 178 with no hearing impairment. The respondents with hearing impairment attended school for hearing-impaired children. Some of the respondents with hearing impairment live in abroad school and some with their families. As an instrument, the authors used a scale for assessing behavioral disorders (Dimoski, 2004), which was filled by the specialists working in the institutions for children and youth with hearing impairments. The survey did not show statistically significant differences in the presence of behavioral disorders in the sample without hearing impairment and the sample of individuals with hearing impairment. However, the results showed that the children with hearing impairment showed significantly greater degree of two indicators of behavioral disorders - the tendency to steal ($t = -3.18$, $p = 0.002$) and extortion of money or benefit from the younger or weaker ($t = -2.07$, $p = 0.039$). This paper also deals with correlates of behavioral disorders in all patients (sex, age, academic achievement, socio-economic status) and with connection to the onset, severity of hearing impairment and type of accommodation (boarding or family) in the group of patients with hearing impairment. The male respondents ($t = 3:07$, $p = 0.003$) with lower school achievement ($F = 11.219$, $p = 0.000$) have more evident indicators of behavioral disorders. This work has important implications relating to the practice of working with children and youth with hearing impairment. It was recommended to work on prevention of behavioral disorders, and suggested which types of psychosocial interventions for those who express this disorder may be used.

In: Handbook of Hearing Disorders Research
Editor: Charlotte Hailee Atkinson

ISBN: 978-1-63463-654-4

Chapter 1

Effect of Hearing Loss on Traffic Safety and Mobility

Birgitta Thorslund, PhD
The Swedish National Road and Transport Research Institute, Sweden

Abstract

Research into the effect of hearing loss (HL) on traffic safety and mobility is limited and the empirical findings are somewhat inconsistent. HL is one of the most frequent sensory deficits in humans, leading to loss of auditory information, which may affect behavior in traffic situations and might reduce traffic safety and mobility. The prevalence of age-related HL in Europe is roughly 30% for men and 20% for women at the age of 70 years, and 55% for men and 45% for women at the age of 80 years. The prevalence of age-related HL is increasing, and as a consequence the number of road users with HL will also increase.

The aim of this PhD thesis was to investigate traffic safety and mobility for individuals with HL. Three studies were conducted: 1. a questionnaire survey aimed to evaluate differences in choice of transportation that might be related to HL, 2. a driving simulator study that looked into compensatory strategies and evaluated the efficiency of a tactile signal to alert the driver, and 3. a field study to evaluate these effects in real traffic and to evaluate a navigation system with a supportive tactile signal.

The results of the three studies indicate that there are effects of HL on traffic safety and mobility. The effects are relatively small and often bound to driving complexity; but, systematic and consistent in replicated study. Differences in transportation habits related to HL include less likelihood of having a driver's license and a higher valuing of written information, with the latter possibly prioritized before time and safety issues. Moreover, respondents with more HL were less concerned about the effects of HL, which suggests that they might be using compensatory strategies.

In the experimental studies, differences in driving behavior related to HL were bound to driving conditions and occurred when the complexity of the driving task increased. There was also an effect of HL on visual behavior, indicated in the simulator and confirmed in the field study, suggesting that drivers with HL have more active visual behaviors with more frequent glances in the rear-view mirror and a general scanning of the environment before looking away from the road. A tactile signal in the driver seat was found useful in both experimental studies, both for calling for the driver's attention and facilitating navigation using a GPS navigation device.

It was concluded that there are effects of HL on both traffic safety and mobility, consistently pointing toward a generally more cautious driving behavior with the use of both compensatory and coping strategies, which suggests a difference in experienced safety. Compensatory strategies associated with HL include driving at lower speeds and using a more comprehensive visual search behavior. Coping strategies associated with HL include engaging less in distracting activities. Evaluation of the tactile signal suggests that it may make driver assistance systems more accessible, not only to drivers with HL, but to all drivers. At the same time, the systems might become more effective for all users, since visual resources can be more focused on the road, which could increase both traffic safety and mobility in general.

List of Papers

Paper I: Thorslund, B., Peters, B., Lyxell, B., & Lidestam, B. (2013). The Influence of Hearing Loss on Transport Safety and Mobility. *European Transport Research Review*, 5(3), 117-127.

Paper II: Thorslund, B., Peters, B., Lidestam, B., & Lyxell, B. (2013). Cognitive workload and driving behavior in persons with hearing loss. *Submitted to Transportation Research Part F*: *Traffic Psychology and Behaviour,* 21, 113-121.

Paper III: Thorslund, B., Ahlström, C., Peters, B., Eriksson, O., Lyxell, B., & Lidestam, B. (2014, May 29). Cognitive workload and visual behavior in elderly persons with hearing loss. *European Transport Research Review*, published online first, 1-9. doi:10.1007/s12544-014-0139-z

Paper IV: Thorslund, B., Peters, B., Herbert, N., Holmqvist, K., Lidestam, B., Black, A., Lyxell, B. (2013). Hearing loss and a supportive tactile signal in a navigation system: Effects on driving behavior and eye movements. *Journal of Eye Movement Research,* 6(5), 1-9.

List of Abbreviations

ADAS	Advanced driver assistance system
CDT	Clock-drawing test
EF	Executive function
HL	Hearing loss
HMI	Human machine interaction
HRF	Swedish Association for Hard of Hearing People
ICF	International Classification of Functioning, Disability and Health
LTM	Long-term memory
MCZ	Multiple comfort zone model
NH	Normal hearing
OR	Odds ratio
PTA	Pure tone average
RAT	Risk allostasis theory

RHM	Risk homeostasis model
RMM	Risk monitor model
TDH	Task difficult homeostasis
TIPS	Text information processing system
TMT	Trail making test
UFOV	Useful field of view
WHO	World Health Organization
WM	Working memory

Concepts and Definitions

Age-related HL Presbycusis: The most common type of HL typically starting around middle adulthood and then progressing, particularly affecting the high frequency ranges.

Compensatory strategies: Efforts made by the individual (consciously or unconsciously) to maintain a given level of functioning despite decline in, or loss of, previously available resources

Coping strategies: Use of conscious effort to solve personal and interpersonal problems and to seek to master, minimize, or tolerate stress or conflict.

Mobility: The quality or state of being mobile. The ability to move freely.

Older adults: Individuals over 65 years

Introduction

For many people transportation is a part of everyday life and is so established that we do not think about how complex even the simplest task really is. Being a road user demands cognitive skills in order to assemble new information in the traffic environment, apply it to stored knowledge, and make decisions. This thesis examines the travel habits and driving behaviors of individuals with hearing loss (HL) and how cognitive skills interact with their driving behavior. Driving a car is a cognitively initiated and controlled task, and thus one approach to understand driving behavior is to examine how cognitive skills are involved. Cognitive psychology is the area that describes the internal processes involved in making sense of the environment and deciding what action might be appropriate (Eysenck & Keane, 2010; Neisser, 1976).

HL is one of the most frequent sensory deficits in humans, with a prevalence of approximately 10% in the general population in the western world, and it is a common chronic condition among the elderly (Stevens et al., 2013). HL entails a loss of auditory information, which may affect behavior in traffic and might reduce traffic safety. Research into the effect of HL on traffic safety and mobility is limited and the empirical findings are somewhat inconsistent. From a legal perspective, based on this relatively low level of knowledge, HL is not considered an increased traffic safety risk (Englund, 2001; Glad, 1977), and therefore hearing is not required for obtaining a driver's license for passenger cars.

From a safety perspective, some studies suggest an association between HL and increased risks of traffic accidents (Ivers, Mitchell, & Cumming, 1999; Picard et al., 2008). However, other studies show no such relation (Green, McGwin, & Owsley, 2013; McCloskey, Koepsell, Wolf, & Buchner, 1994). Schmolz (1987) examined the importance of hearing for road users and found that HL is associated with a higher degree of inattention. With regard to attention, Hickson et al. (2012) showed that HL in older drivers was associated with poorer driving performance in the presence of distraction, but not without distraction. On the other hand, Picard et al. (2008) suggested that HL leads to a reduction in speeding violations, probably due to self-regulation. In sum, the effect of HL on traffic safety remains mostly unknown, and possibly connected to specific situations; although its associations with attention and driving speed have been shown.

From a mobility perspective, it is possible that of HL leads to self-regulation due to feelings of unsafety. This is an important aspect to consider, because mobility is important for quality of life (Farquhar, 1995), often connected to factors such as psychological well-being and independence (Bonnel, 1999; Fonda, Wallace, & Herzog, 2001; Gabriel & Bowling, 2004; Marottoli et al., 1997), and also associated with higher life satisfaction (Banister & Bowling, 2004; Hakamies-Blomqvist & Wahlström, 1998 Gagliardi, Marcellini, Papa, Giuli, & Mollenkopf, 2010).

Physiologically, disruption of any part along the auditory pathway (central to peripheral) may lead to HL and there are two main diagnoses. Problems in the outer ear (such as blockage of the ear canal) or middle ear (such as ossicular chain discontinuity) cause conductive hearing loss, and problems in the inner ear (such as loss of outer or inner hair cells in the cochlea) or problems in the auditory nerve leading to the central auditory pathway (such as auditory neuropathy) can result in sensorineural HL (Arlinger, 2007).

This thesis is focused on age-related HL, also known as presbycusis. This is the most common type of HL typically starting around middle adulthood and progressing, affecting the high frequency ranges particularly (Pearson et al., 1995; Schneider, Pichora-Fuller, & Daneman, 2010) and inducing distortion (Moore, 1995). The prevalence of age-related HL in Europe is roughly 30% for men and 20% for women at the age of 70 years, and 55% for men and 45% for women at the age of 80 years (Roth, Hanebuth, & Probst, 2001). The prevalence of age-related HL is increasing, due to populations becoming progressively older and thus presenting symptoms of reduced sensory function. A consequence of the increasing prevalence of HL is that the number of road users (not only drivers) with HL will also increase. This certainly leads to an increased need of knowledge about these individuals with regard to traffic safety and mobility.

Hearing is important for our sense of spatial orientation and temporal resolution and thus of high relevance for traffic safety. Sounds behind us provide information about events that it not possible to see and we receive information about positions and distances. Most frequency spectra of exterior tires or road noise display a prominent peak in the range of 700–1300 Hz (Sandberg, 2003). Since the noise from cars driving on roads is mainly in low frequencies, i.e. with low-pitched sounds (Wu, Stangl, Bentler, & Stanziola, 2013), individuals with presbycusis should be able to hear these specific sounds rather well. However, there might be other vital auditory input in high frequencies (e.g. a bicycle bell can be hard to hear for a pedestrian), which is partly or totally missed, and may therefore lead to loss of critical information for the listener. Distortion leads to increased difficulties in hearing masked sounds, in other words low frequency traffic noise can mask high frequency sounds. Research on effective siren characteristics suggest either a sufficiently loud, wide frequency spectrum (1-4 kHz) to overcome masking noise (De Lorenzo & Eilers, 1991; Catchpole & McKeown,

2007) or sirens that broadcast low frequencies so that the siren sound can penetrate into vehicle cabins (Howard et al., 2011). Furthermore, the use of in-vehicle systems for information, support, and navigation is rapidly increasing. These systems often use auditory signals that may not be accessible to drivers with HL. Thus, investigating other modalities such as light or vibration should be considered to also make these systems accessible to drivers with HL.

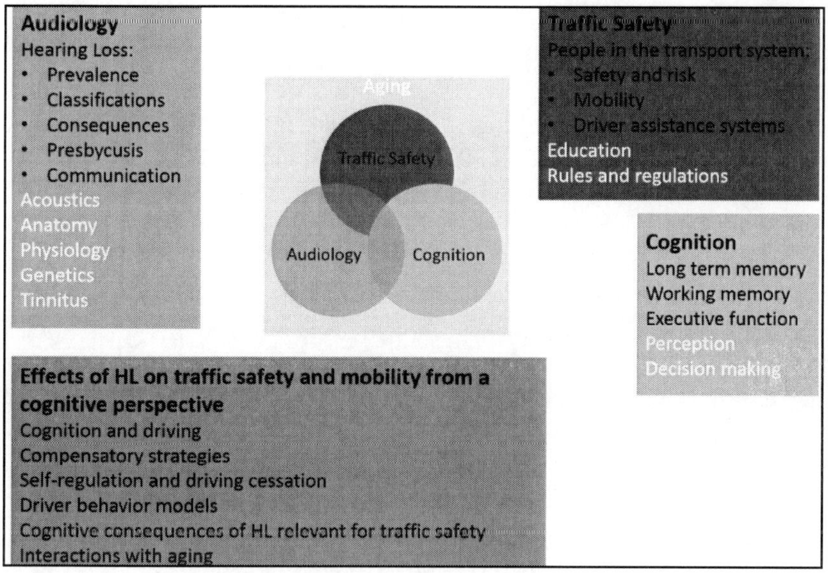

Figure 1. Overview of the thesis. The three main topics are Traffic Safety, Audiology and Cognition. These are presented and discussed separately, in relation to each other and in relation to age. Concepts included in the thesis are listed in black and terms excluded or mentioned only briefly are listed in white.

In the present thesis, traffic safety and mobility for individuals with HL is examined from the perspective of cognitive psychology. That is, how different cognitive skills in combination with HL affect traffic safety and mobility. Focus is on the intersection between three research areas: *audiology*, *cognition,* and *traffic safety*. The background and central expressions of these areas and their interrelations with each other and with age are presented in the following chapters. Figure 1 presents an overview of the thesis in terms of what is covered or excluded in each area, as well as in the intersection between them.

Hearing Loss

The International Classification of Functioning, Disability and Health (ICF) suggested by the World Health Organization (WHO) is a framework based on the biopsychosocial model that describes the consequences of a particular health condition or disability in terms of various levels of disablement and functioning (WHO, 2001). These may include body functions on the organic level, activities on the personal level, and participation on the social level. These levels also interact with each other and may be further influenced by personal and environmental factors. Thus, it is important to understand the consequences of a particular health condition or disability from multiple perspectives (Rimmer, 2006).

According to the ICF, functioning and disability are typically conceptualized as a complex interaction between an individual's health condition, contextual factors of the environment, and personal factors (WHO, 2001). The consequences of HL include the inability to interpret speech sounds, often producing a reduced ability to communicate, delay in language acquisition in children, economic and educational disadvantage, social isolation, and stigmatization. This may also be worsened by some medical conditions such as diabetes (Mathers, Smith, & Concha, 2003).

The degree of HL is categorized according to the better ear hearing level averaged over the frequencies of 0.5, 1, 2, and 4 kHz and divided into mild (26-40 dB), moderate (41-60 dB), severe (61-80 dB), and profound (> 80 dB) (Mathers, et al., 2003). Individuals with a HL of 95 dB or more are commonly referred to as deaf.

Age-related HL, the focus of this thesis, originates with the deterioration of auditory function and is part of normal aging, usually starting in the middle adulthood (Pearson et al., 1995; Schneider, Pichora-Fuller, & Daneman, 2010). Outer hair-cell damage, degeneration of the stria vascularis (producing endocochlear potential) and the auditory nerve are the main causes (Pichora-Fuller & Singh, 2006), and auditory processes, such as temporal resolution and duration discrimination, are negatively affected (Fitzgibbons & Gordon-Salant, 2010; Saremi & Stenfelt, 2013).

Assessment of Hearing Ability

Assessment of hearing ability is performed either psychoacoustically with an active listener (e.g., tone audiometry) or by objective methods using a physiological reaction such as electro-physical methods or otoacoustic emissions (Arlinger, 2007). Pure-tone average (PTA) is a common hearing test, relying on a patient's response to pure-tone stimuli. With PTA both air and bone conduction can be tested thus, enabling the determination of degree, type, and configuration of HL in an individual. Test frequencies begin at 1000 Hz and include at a minimum octave steps up to 8000 Hz and down to 125 Hz. Often 750, 1500, 3000, and 6000 Hz are also included. Figure 2 shows results from a PTA marked in an audiogram with test frequencies on the horizontal axis and hearing thresholds on the vertical.

Cognition

Cognitive psychology is a necessary part for explaining human behavior. The cognitive approach is used to explain the mental processes essential for our ability to perceive and attend to, as well as memorize and communicate with, the world around us. These cognitive processes also are fundamental for our language perception, production and use, thinking, and problem solving (Eysenck & Keane, 2010). The concept 'attention' is successively being replaced by executive functions (EFs), which are defined as a high-level process with the main obligation of adapting to new and complex situations (Diamond, 2013; Eysenck & Keane, 2010). Working memory (WM) and long-term memory (LTM) are 2 separate memory systems, which according to Baddeley (2012) are linked together by an episodic buffer working as an interface between the 2 memory systems. In order to understand the possible cognitive consequences of HL relevant for traffic safety it is important to understand both cognitive consequences of HL and road user behavior.

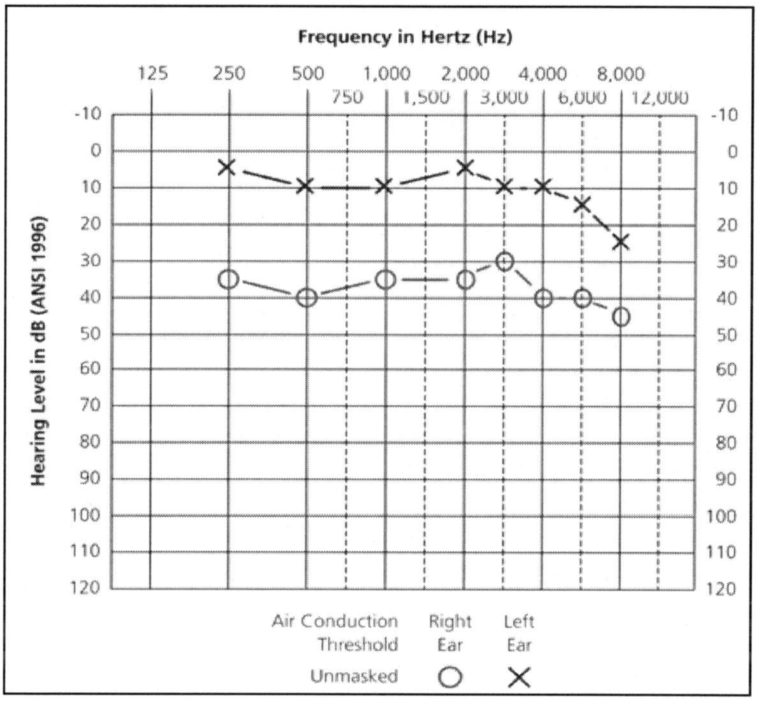

Figure 2. An audiogram presenting hearing thresholds from a PTA (air conduction).

The main focus in the present thesis is on car drivers with age- related HL. WM, LTM and EFs are involved since previous research has shown the effects of age (e.g., McDowd & Shaw, 2000; Verhaeghen et al., 2003) and HL (e.g., Andersson & Lyxell 1999; Lin et al., 2011, 2013; Rönnberg et al., 2011) on these systems. Cognitive factors such as perception and decision making is not actively examined even though effects of aging have been observed in previous studies (e.g., Johnson, 1989; Kennedy, Taylor, Reade, & Yesavage, 2010). The reason for this is the limited knowledge in this area and there is a need for constraints to be able to focus on some specific issues.

Working Memory

WM refers to a memory system with a limited capacity, and that serves to simultaneously store and process new information over a short period of time (Daneman & Carpenter, 1980; Daneman & Merikle, 1996; Miyake & Shah, 1999; Baddeley, 2012). WM is necessary in daily life in that it helps us keep things in mind when approaching a task. For example, remembering what to write down once we have found the piece of paper and a pencil or remembering what we have read once we get to the end of the sentence. In the multicomponent model of WM (Baddeley, 2012; Repovs & Baddeley, 2006) there are 4 components, each serving a specific purpose. A central executive serves as a modality independent control system, which directs and divides attention between tasks. It is involved whenever manipulation within WM is required (Repovs & Baddeley, 2006). This means the central executive controls the function of the subordinate storage components, namely: the phonological loop (dealing with language-based verbal information); the visuospatial sketchpad (processing visuospatial information); and the episodic buffer (providing a link between new and old information) (Repovs & Baddeley, 2006).

The phonological loop comprises 2 components: a passive phonological store, which holds memory traces, like speech, in acoustic or phonological form for a few seconds; and an articulatory rehearsal process linked to speech production, recoding information from other modalities (Repovs & Baddeley, 2006). According to this words and letters presented auditorily are processed differently from those presented visually. Auditory sensations have direct access to the phonological store, regardless of whether the articulatory control process is used. In contrast visual presentation of words and letters only produces indirect access through sub-vocal articulation (Baddeley, 2012; Eysenck & Keane, 2010).

The visuospatial sketchpad is dedicated to the storage and manipulation of visual and spatial information. The fourth component is the episodic buffer, which serves as an interface for binding information from different sensory sources, the other 2 subsidiary systems, and LTM. The episodic buffer also serves as an interface between perception and LTM, where the phonological and semantic representations in the lexicon are stored (Baddeley, 1983; Repovs & Baddeley, 2006). WM capacity is related to performance in most other complex cognitive tasks such as reading comprehension and problem solving (Conway, Kane & Engle, 2003). WM capacity is one reflection of individual differences in the ability to focus and maintain attention, specifically when other events are serving to capture one's attention (Kane & Engle, 2002).

In sum, WM is the ability to temporarily hold information, manipulate and use this for a special cause over a short period of time. One example from a traffic situation is a road user (driver, pedestrian or cyclist) who is about to cross the street. They must keep track of the positions of the other road users and use this information to calculate when to cross.

Long-term Memory

LTM is a memory system where information is stored for long periods of time and remains indefinitely. In this system, declarative memory includes episodic memory and semantic memory, while non-declarative memory is divided into repetition priming and procedural memory (Eysenck & Keane, 2010). Episodic memory is the memory of personal events (e.g., times, places, associated emotions, and other contextual knowledge) that can be explicitly stated, which is used when driving to a specific known place. The semantic LTM includes general knowledge about the world (e.g., languages, game rules, names of capital cities, authors of books, traffic rules) that the individual shares with others. The perceptual representation system recognizes items and terms, permitting rapid identification of previously encountered stimulants (perceptual or conceptual). As the name implies, procedural memory stores information on how to perform certain procedures such as walking, riding a bike and maneuvering a car (Eysenck & Keane, 2010).

Executive Functions

EFs are a set of mental processes that help us stay focused on what we are supposed to focus on (Diamond, 2013). EFs is a relatively new concept in the sense that we can relate to it more theoretically today than previously. EFs are used to perform activities such as planning, organizing, making, and using strategies, paying attention to and remembering details, and managing time and space. EFs make it possible to play with ideas, take the time to think before acting, meet novel, unanticipated challenges, resist temptations, and stay focused (Diamond, 2013). Miyake et al. (2000) defined shifting, updating and inhibiting as 3 specifically important EFs, correlated but separable. Shifting was defined by Monsell (1996) as responsible for attentional or task shifting. Updating monitors and codes incoming information according to relevance for the current task. This manipulation, instead of just storing, was described as the most important function of the updating function by Morris and Jones (1990). Miyake defined inhibition as the possibility of deliberately stopping dominant, automatic or powerful reactions and necessary to minimize distraction effects (Miyake et al., 2000).

Researchers have argued that WM capacity reflects the efficiency of EFs, especially the ability to maintain a few task-relevant representations and neglecting irrelevant information (Engle, Tuholski, Laughlin, & Conway, 1999). According to Diamond (2013), the main EFs are: inhibition, which is divided into response inhibition (self-control-resisting temptations and resisting acting impulsively) and interference control (selective attention and cognitive inhibition); WM; and cognitive flexibility (including creatively thinking outside the box, seeing anything from different perspectives, and quickly and flexibly adapting to changed circumstances).

In sum, EFs are essential in helping us in our daily life. They help us stay focused on what we are doing by updating us with relevant information and neglecting unrelated information. EFs also help us shift between tasks and think before acting, which is essential for driving a car. For example, visualization of consequences, analysis of information, and judgment of time, distance and power are necessary to be able to drive a car safely.

Assessment of Cognitive Ability

Cognitive decline is, just like HL, a part of normal aging and also related to HL (Baltes & Lindenberger, 1997; Rönnberg et al., 2011; Valentijn, van Boxtel, & van Hooren, 2005). Therefore, it is important to control for differences in cognitive abilities when comparing driving performance between a group with HL and a group with NH. This can be accomplished by cognitive testing.

WM Capacity

There are several tests designed to evaluate WM capacity. A commonly used measure is a dual-task paradigm combining a memory span measure with a concurring processing task. Daneman and Carpenter (1980) invented the first version of this kind of task, called the "reading span test". In their test participants read a number of sentences (usually between 2-6) and tried to remember the last word of each sentence. At the end of the list of sentences, they tried to repeat back the words in the correct order. Individual WM capacity, as measured by the reading span test (Andersson, Lyxell, Rönnberg, & Spens, 2001; Daneman & Carpenter, 1980; Rönnberg, 1990), has shown to account for 40% of the inter-individual variance of speech recognition in noise among participants with similar levels of HL (Lunner, 2003).

Impairments in visuospatial ability (measured by, for example, copying the wire cube, pentagons, drawing a clock face) are good markers of increased driving risk (Kipps & Hodges, 2005). The clock drawing test (CDT) is a simple tool that is used to screen people for signs of neurological problems such as Alzheimer's and other dementias. CDT assesses primarily EFs by letting the participant draw a clock with hands pointing at a specific time.

TIPS (Text Information Processing System, Ausmeel, 1988), is a cognitive test platform developed according to established cognitive models of WM, phonological and lexical ability (see Baddeley, 2012; Abreu, Gathercole, & Martin, 2011; Shah & Miyake, 1996). The battery intends to measure WM capacity, phonological abilities and lexical abilities, and thus includes several tests for each of these cognitive aspects. A shorter computer-based version of TIPS was developed for use in clinics. Both this and TIPS have been used in a large number of studies (e.g., Hällgren, Larsby, Lyxell, & Arlinger, 2001, Bergemalm, Hennerdal, Persson, Lyxell, & Borg, 2009; Lidestam, Lyxell, & Andersson, 1999; Hua, 2014). The reading span test aims to measure the WM capacity. Two tests include reaction time measure of phonological ability (deciding whether 2 letters are identical and deciding whether 2 words rhyme).

Processing Speed, Divided Attention, Selective Attention

Skills measured by Useful Field of View (UFOV) are used during driving (Ball & Owsley, 1993), and the test is intended to be indicative of accident risk in the older population (Ball, Owsley, Sloane, Roenker, & Bruni, 1993; Owsley et al., 1998). In the first subtest, measuring processing speed, the participant is asked to identify which vehicle (car or truck) is displayed on the screen for a short time. In the second subtest, evaluating divided attention, the participant should, in addition to the first task, localize a car placed in the periphery on the screen. The third subtest, assessing selective attention, is identical to subtest 2 but with the rest of the screen filled with distracting triangles.

The trail-making test (TMT) assesses visual search, processing speed and mental flexibility (Reitan, 1986). Part A consists of targets marked with numbers, which are connected in numerical order, and part B are targets marked with both numbers and letters, which are connected in a combined numerical and alphabetical order such as 1-A-2-B-3-C and so on. On a computerized version of TMT developed by Summala et al. (2008), the target locations are fixed on the screen but the content, that is numbers or letters, are either the same (fixed) or randomly changed after each tap on a touch screen instead of the traditional pen and paper version.

Hearing Loss, Cognition and Aging

Commonly, when talking about older people, older adults and elderly, this refers to individuals over the age of 65 (Gordon-Salant, 2005; Gorman, 1999; Roebuck, 1979). This also applies for this present thesis. Numerous studies have shown that there is a correlation between HL and cognitive decline in old age (Granick, Kleban, & Weiss, 1976; Thomas, Hunt, Garry, Hood, Goodwin, & Goodwin, 1983; Lindenberger & Baltes, 1994; Baltes &

Lindenberger, 1997; Li & Lindenberger, 2002; Lin, Ferrucci, Metter, An, Zonderman, & Resnick, 2011; Rönnberg et al., 2011), which will be presented more specifically in a subsequent section.

Because age-related HL is the most common type (Roth, Hanebuth, & Probst, 2001; WHO, 2001), it is important to understand other consequences of normal aging, which more or less affect or are affected by HL. For example, the deterioration of auditory functions such as like speech understanding is worsened by age-related changes in the cognitive system (Grady, 2012; Rönnlund, Nyberg, Bäckman, & Nilsson, 2005). Older adults with NH have also shown more difficulties with speech recognition than younger individuals with NH (Frisina & Frisina, 1997; Gordon-Salant, 2005), which can, for example, affect the possibility of using auditory-based driver assistance systems.

Cognitive Consequences of Aging

Aging is associated with the decline in the control processes involved in coordinating distinct tasks such as reaction times, WM tasks, tests of episodic memory, tests of spatial and reasoning abilities, mental rotation, and visual search performance (McDowd & Shaw, 2000; Verhaeghen et al., 2003). However, on specific vocabulary tests, no effects of age have been shown, for example by Elliott et al. (2003) using the Wechsler Adult Intelligence Scale Vocabulary subtest (Jastak & Jastak, 1964) and by Bowles and Salthouse (2009) using multiple-choice synonyms, multiple-choice antonyms and produce-the-definition.

The effects of aging have also been demonstrated when switching between specific tasks (e.g., switching between responding to color or form and responding only to color, Mayr et al., 2001; Verhaeghen et al. 2005), and are also related to attention (Craik & Salthouse, 2000; Phillips & Lesperance, 2003). Slower cognitive processing is also associated with aging (Cerella, 1990; Salthouse, 1996) and it is estimated that processing takes 1.5-2 times longer in older than in younger adults (Cerella, 1990). This affects most age related declines in performing complex cognitive tasks such as problem solving, reasoning and language comprehension (Salthouse, 1996; Verhaegen et al., 2003).

Aging is also associated with reductions in WM for both processing (van der Linden et al., 1994, 1999; Bopp & Verhaeghen, 2005) and capacity (Bopp & Verhaeghen, 2005; Salthouse & Babcock, 1991). Specifically, the episodic memory of LTM is negatively affected by age while semantic memory remains relatively stable or may even increase, and on the non-declarative memory no conclusive aging effect has been shown (Brickman & Stern, 2009).

Some of these age-related cognitive declines can be of major importance for safe mobility (e.g., reaction times, visual search performance, processing speed, problem solving), specifically for driving, which according to Groeger (2000) is one of the most complex and safety critical everyday tasks in modern society.

Cognitive Consequences of HL

Specific and general effects of HL on cognitive functions have been demonstrated (e.g., Andersson, 2002, Lin et al., 2011, Rönnberg et al., 2011). For example, a relationship between severe to profound HL and deficiency in certain aspects of phonological processing has been demonstrated and suggested to come from a gradual loss of specificity of phonological representations (Andersson, 2002; Andersson & Lyxell 1999; Lyxell, Andersson, Borg, & Ohlson 2003; Rönnberg et al., 2011; Classon, 2013). Andersson (2002) concluded that specific aspects of the phonological system deteriorate in the HL population as a function of auditory deprivation. In particular, the phonological representations are impaired and this impairment also affects the ability to rapidly perform phonological operations.

HL has been demonstrated as independently associated with accelerated cognitive decline (30-40%) and incident cognitive impairment (24%) among older adults during a six-year period. (Lin et al., 2011). These effects have been shown with the Modified Mini-Mental State test (Teng & Chui, 1987), which is a verbal cognitive test, as well as with a non-verbal cognitive test (called Digit Symbol Substitution, Wechsler, 1981), in both cross-sectional and prospective studies (Valentijn et al., 2005; Peters, Potter, & Scholer, 1988). Specifically, verbal tests have shown the relationship between HL and cognitive decline more extensively than non-verbal tests (Granick et al., 1976; Thomas et al., 1983).

The more general effects of HL on cognitive functions may affect traffic safety more and are in line with Baddeley (2012), who found that articulatory suppression leads to WM decline. Prospective studies have found accelerated cognitive decline and increased risk of dementia and Alzheimer's in individuals with HL (Lin et al., 2011, 2013). Cross-sectional studies have shown that HL is associated with lower performance in tests of EFs and free recall (Lin, 2011) and has a negative effect on episodic and semantic LTM (Rönnberg et al., 2011). With a decline in WM, EFs and LTM, it might, for example, be more difficult to stay focused on the driving task, keep track of the surrounding traffic or to remember traffic rules.

Another aspect worth considering is cognitive fatigue, due to higher effort in listening, leading to decreased cognitive capacity. This effect has been shown on both young and adult listeners with HL (Arlinger, 2003; Hicks & Tharpe, 2002; Tun, McCoy, & Wingfield, 2009). In addition, several studies have shown that hearing aids do not fully restore speech difficulties of individuals with HL (e.g., Dimitrijevic et al., 2004; Moradi, Lidestam, Hällgren, & Rönnberg, 2014; Nakeva von Mentzer, 2014), which made perceiving speech stimuli cognitively demanding (Moradi et al., 2014; Rönnberg et al., 2013).

This cognitively demanding processing of speech stimuli may increase fatigue in individuals with HL during conversations with their partners while they are driving. Cognitive fatigue could, among other things, lead to decreased attention and thus be relevant to traffic safety. Moreover, mobility might be affected if cognitive fatigue leads to decreased driving.

Furthermore, dual sensory decline (hearing and vision) is associated with cognitive decline and for a functional decline on everyday activities over a period of 4 years (Lin, Guttierrez, & Stone et al., 2004). Thus, research questions with regard to age-related HL and traffic safety require the combined study of several factors associated with declines due to aging.

In sum, specific cognitive declines of HL have been demonstrated and include, for example, phonological deficiencies (processing and representation) as a consequence of less auditory stimulation (specificity of phonological representations). Traffic safety might be affected due to a decline in WM, EFs and LTM, which can lead to difficulties to stay focused on the driving task, keep track of the traffic around or to remember traffic rules. Also, cognitive fatigue could lead to decrease in attention and thus be of relevance for traffic safety.

Cognition and Traffic Safety

Groeger (2000) described driving a car as one of the most complex and safety critical daily tasks in modern society (Groeger, 2000). Driving is a cognitively motivated and controlled task. When demands are high, driving is carried out in a force-paced way, while when the demands are low, in a more self-paced way (Peters & Nilsson, 2006). Thus, workload is an aspect of driving that should be considered, and in this thesis the term *cognitive workload* is used, when others might be using *mental workload.* De Waard (1996) defined driver workload as the individual reaction to driving task demand and further refers to Rouse et al., who defined experienced load, which is not only task-specific but also person-specific. (Rouse Edwards, & Hammer, 1993).

More specifically, workload is the specification of the amount of information processing capacity that is used for task performance. Therefore, workload depends on the individual, and owing to the interaction between operator and task structure the same task demands do not result in an equal level of workload for all individuals (de Waard, 1996).

Directly related to driving task demand is task complexity. According to de Waard (1996), complexity increases with an increase in the number of stages of processing that are required to perform a task. Task demand and complexity are mainly external, but both depend on subjective goals set for task performance. Difficulty of a task is related to the processing effort that is required by the individual for task performance, and is dependent on context, state, capacity, and strategy or policy of allocation of resources (de Waard, 1996).

Driving effort is dynamic, as the cognitive demands can change back and forth from very low to extremely high, sometimes within fractions of a second (Michon, 1985; Peters & Nilsson, 2006). Among the factors determining the driving task demand, of which the driver has immediate and direct control, driving speed is the most significant (Fuller, 2005). It has been demonstrated that when a threshold of a certain preferred driving speed is exceeded, experienced task difficulty, effort and feeling of risk is affected (Lewis-Evans, 2011).

In sum, driver workload is the individual reaction to driving task demand, which is directly related to task complexity. Task demand and complexity changes back and forth due to external circumstances and subjective goals, which makes the driving task and driver workload very dynamic. Feelings of risk arise when the task complexity goes above a certain threshold.

Driver Behavior Models

An advance within traffic behavioral research has been the increased understanding of the driving task from a cognitive perspective, and consequently the skills needed for carrying out this task successfully and safely. Since perceptual and psychomotor abilities are essential to model driving behavior, driving can be viewed as a cognitive task of control in a context perceived through the senses and manipulated with control actions based on unconscious (automated) or conscious decisions (Peters & Nilsson, 2006).

Carsten (2007) distinguishes between 2 broad types of driver models. The first type is descriptive of parts or the whole of a driving task in terms of *what the driver has to do* and includes, for example, task models (Michon, 1985; McKnight & Adams, 1970), adaptive control models (McRuer et al., 1977; Hollnagel et al., 2003), and production models (Michon, 1985). Michon (1985) described driving a car as a complex task with processes at a minimum of 3 hierarchical levels. At the top level, the strategic level, strategic decisions are made such as the choice of means of transport, setting of a route goal, and route-choice while driving. At the intermediate level, the maneuvering level, reactions to local situations, including reactions to the behavior of other traffic participants, take place. Basic vehicle-control processes, such as lateral-position control, occur at the lowest level, the control level. At this level automatic processes occur, while at higher levels higher controlled processing is required.

The second type is motivational models, aiming to describe *how the driver manages task difficulty*. In contrast to the descriptive models, sometimes being merely descriptive or analytical, motivational models attempt to explain which psychological factors affect driver behavior and why drivers make certain decisions (Michon, 1985).

According to Ranney (1994), errors associated with the variability of human behavior may be more important to roadway crash causation than systematic errors, which are attributable to the known limits of the human information-processing system. Furthermore, given the ever-increasing variety of driving situations, including changes in the driving task associated with different technologies, and the corresponding variety of skills and abilities required, Ranney (1994) claimed it unlikely that a comprehensive model of driver behavior will ever be feasible.

For the purpose of this thesis, we expect that differences related to HL are not as likely to occur in terms of what the driver has to do, but rather may occur in the management of task difficulty and when making certain decisions. Therefore, motivational driver behavior models will be presented and discussed in more detail from the HL perspective.

Motivational Models

The most well-known motivational model is Wilde's (1982) Risk Homeostatis Model (RHM), introducing the notion of driver capability affecting risk (Carsten, 2007). Wilde proposed that there is a preferred target level of risk of being involved in an accident that drivers seek to maintain. Fuller and Santos (2002) proposed the Task Difficult Homeostasis (TDH) (see also Fuller, 2005, 2007; Fuller et al., 2008; Fuller, McHugh et al., 2008), stating that people have a set range of experienced task difficulty at which they prefer to operate. TDH was then re-conceptualized into Risk Allostasis Theory (RAT), where the acceptable range of task difficulty is accompanied by and essentially interchangeable with a range of preferred feeling of risk (Fuller, 2008; Fuller, 2011).

The Risk Monitor Model (RMM) (Vaa et al., 2000; Vaa, 2003, 2007, 2011) suggests that all individuals have a drive to maintain or obtain a target best feeling, which is variable in both its value and the type of feeling, however, including, for example: tension or anxiety, arousal, sensation, pleasure, relaxation, difficulty avoidance, compliance, and non-compliance (Vaa, 2007).

The Multiple Comfort Zone model (MCZ) by Summala (2005) is an evolution of the earlier zero-risk theory (Näätänen & Summala, 1974). Being a motivational model it views a driver's excitatory motives, personality and driving goals as prevailing factors. These motives interact with the road system and push drivers toward changing their behavior to satisfy their driving goals, for example by increasing speed to arrive at a destination on time (Summala, 2005; Summala, 2007).

What the presented motivational models all have in common is the level of risk, and it is suggested that the driver aims at maintaining this level. Whether drivers with HL are at higher risk than NH drivers or not is uncertain since there are studies suggesting connections between HL and higher risks of traffic accidents (Ivers, Mitchell, & Cumming, 1999; Picard et al., 2008) and also research where no such relationship has been found (Green, McGwin, & Owsley, 2013; McCloskey, Koepsell, Wolf, & Buchner, 1994). However, if there is a difference in risk related to HL there should, according to the motivational models, also be a different level of risk in which the drivers with HL aim to maintain. This could be driving at a lower speed, for example.

Lewis-Evans (2012) experimentally tested 4 motivational models of driver behavior: TDH, RAT, RMM, and the MCZ (Summala, 2005; Summala, 2007). He concluded that the speed is not solely a conscious choice but handled, at least at some difficulty level, by automatic processes, and that the existence of these processes can be inferred when the cognitive capability of drivers is put to the test. Furthermore, results from the experiments supported the idea of a threshold to account for the perception of subjective variables such as task difficulty, effort, comfort, crash risk, and feeling of risk. For predicting difficulty of the task, the variables that the participants were most sensitive to changes in were speed and following distance. Lewis-Evans (2012) claims that these findings support models such as the MCZ (Summala, 2005; Summala, 2007) due to the reliance of this model on actual performance measures in driving such as time to line crossing or time to collision.

In line with Lewis-Evans' findings are the results from Lidestam, Lundqvist and Rönnberg (2010), who tested the external validity of theoretical driver behavior models by letting traffic inspectors rate the importance of theoretical concepts found in research literature on risk awareness. It was revealed that visual search was the most important concept, and that the assessment of risk awareness can be conceptualized as assessment of lower-order (maneuvering and position, cf. Michon's control level) and higher-order (attention, traffic behavior and speed, cf. Michon's manoeuver level) cognitive functions.

In sum, according to motivational driver behavior models, drivers aim to maintain a preferred level of risk. The results in Lewis-Evans (2012) with regard to speed and following distance suggest time-based safety margins as relevant measures of this individual level of risk, and visual search is proposed as a valid indicator of risk awareness (Lidestam et al., 2010). This is all in line with Gibson and Crooks' very first model of driver behavior: field of safe travel (Gibson & Crooks, 1938). All of this is relevant for understanding the effect of HL on driving behavior and for the evaluation of driver support systems. Recurring in the models is the driving speed, and several studies have linked speed perception to the amount of noise in car cabins or to the driving sound (Evans, 1970; Ohta & Komatsu, 1991). Thus, speed might be perceived differently by drivers with hearing loss, due to a reduced sensitivity to sounds.

Traffic Safety

One goal of traffic research should be to provide the safest possible mobility for all road users, regardless of their levels or types of abilities or disabilities. In all motivational models presented above, drivers aim to maintain a preferred level of risk, above a certain threshold. Whether drivers with HL are at higher risk than NH drivers is uncertain because previous findings are contradictory. For example, some studies found increased risk for drivers with HL (Ivers, Mitchell, & Cumming, 1999; Picard et al., 2008), while others did not (Green, McGwin, & Owsley, 2013; McCloskey, Koepsell, Wolf, & Buchner, 1994).

According to Rumar (1988), there is always a risk in being mobile, and he divided risk into statistical (objective) risk and experienced (also called subjective or perceived) risk. For drivers with HL, research results are limited and rather contradictory on objective risk, and we found no results on subjective risk in our extensive literature surveys. Thus, it might be that drivers with HL can experience a subjective risk even if there is no objective risk. Research results so far do not identify clearly increased objective or subjective risks for drivers with HL, but this might be due to lack of knowledge. Therefore, there may be no increased risk at all for drivers with HL; there might be a small and unimportant risk; or there could be an important increased risk research has yet to reveal.

The level of knowledge on the relationship between HL and statistical traffic safety is relatively low and too inconsistent to draw any conclusions. Crash data have shown that drivers with HL are at higher risks of traffic accidents (Ivers, Mitchell, & Cumming, 1999; Picard et al., 2008). However, there is also research on crash data and medical record data where such relationships have not been found (Green, 2013; McCloskey, Koepsell, Wolf, & Buchner, 1994). On the effect of HL on subjective traffic safety the literature is even scarcer. Lundälv (2004) found that adult pedestrians and cyclists with moderate HL had no self-reported experiences of feeling insecure in the traffic environment; however, he also suggested that these individuals are at higher risk of being injured by a vehicle because they report that they find it difficult to identify the direction sounds come from.

While traffic safety and mobility for drivers with HL is almost unexplored, the research literature regarding older drivers is relatively extensive. With age-related HL being the most common type (Roth, Hanebuth, & Probst, 2001; WHO, 2001), the effects of age are very relevant and will be discussed further in the following sections, along with the possible effects of HL.

Mobility and Quality of Life

Transportation is a part of everyday life and may be necessary for participation in activities and social life. Several studies suggest that travel habits will further increase for older adults in the future (Dillén, Schmidt, & Jarlebring, 2005; Hausten et al., 2013; Hjorthol, Levin, & Sirén, 2010) and this is explained by attitudinal effects (higher mobility needs, more active lifestyles), improved physical possibilities (fitness and health conditions), and cohort effects (being born at about the same time, exposed to the same events in society, and influenced by the same demographic trends and thus having similar experiences; Haustein, 2013).

In this thesis, mobility refers to the quality or state of being mobile - the ability to move freely. The ICF model includes mobility in activity and participation. Several studies have proven that limitation of activities increase with the degree of HL (Gopinath, Schneider, Hickson et al., 2012; Grue et al., 2009; Wallhagen et al., 2001; Schneider et al., 2010). HL has also been found to affect instrumental activities such as talking on the telephone or using public transportation more than daily activities such as getting dressed or eating (Gopinath, Schneider, McMahon, et al., 2012).

Car access is associated with better health and well-being among the elderly (Ellaway, Macintyre, Hiscock, & Kearns, 2003; Macintyre, Hiscock, Kearns, & Ellaway, 2001). By enabling older people with physical limitations to still live independently and to participate in normal daily activities, the car can act as a compensational tool for functional limitations (Sirén & Hakamies-Blomqvist, 2004, 2009). According to Köpke, Deubel, Engeln and Schlag (1999), car availability and car use are related to positive self-perception in older people, and research suggests driving cessation may be a risk factor for a depressive development (Fonda, Wallace, & Herzog 2001; Marottoli et al., 1997). With age-related HL being the most common type of HL (Pearson et al., 1995; Schneider, Pichora-Fuller, & Daneman, 2010) and with increasing travel habits among older adults (and the gap between actual mobility and desirable mobility), it is important to understand the effect of HL on mobility.

Self-regulation of driving usually refers to the voluntary reduction or avoidance of certain (typically challenging or demanding) driving situations (Haustein, 2013). This could also be a way of maintaining the level of risk by not exposing oneself to specific traffic situations. Factors found to be associated with self-regulation of driving are functional decline, and increasing cognitive and visual restrictions (Ball et al., 1998; Charlton, Oxley, Fildes, Oxley, & Newstead, 2003; Holland & Rabbit, 1992), and one's perceived driving skills (Gabaude, Marquié, & Obriot-Claudel, 2010; Rimmö & Hakamies-Blomqvist, 2002).

The most common medical conditions affecting driving cessation include sensory problems, cognitive impairment, stroke, cardiovascular, and other heart conditions, diabetes, and physical mobility and activity problems (Brayne et al., 2000; Dellinger, Kresnow, White, & Sehgal 2004; Forrest, Bunker, Songer, Cohen, & Cauley, 1997; Hakamies-Blomqvist & Wahlström, 1998). Edwards et al. (2009) indicated that driving cessation is associated with declines in physical and social functioning, as well as in general health (Edwards, Lunsman, Perkins, Rebok, & Roth, 2009).

In sum, various age-related declines are associated with self-regulation and driving cessation. Because car access is associated with better health among the elderly, it is important to assist driving for older adults when possible. One way of achieving this is to ensure that driver assistance systems are also accessible for drivers with HL.

Effects of Aging on Driving Behavior

Factors associated with old age and that have a negative impact on the ability to drive include impaired perceptual abilities, memory decline, reduction in the ability to sustain and switch attention, and mobility constraints (Groeger, 2000). However, aging is usually a gradual process and while some skills deteriorate with increasing age, others (more strategic) are used more with increasing age (Haustein, 2013).

As car drivers, older persons perceive certain driving situations and conditions as demanding and potentially dangerous. These include driving in specific weather conditions (e.g., fog, rain or a storm), when feeling physically unwell or excited, in high traffic density, on specific road types (e.g., motorways or highways), on roads with certain characteristics (e.g., signals, traffic lights, curves, roundabouts), and in response to others' driving behaviors (e.g., tailgating) (Jansen et al., 2001; Sullivan, Smith, Horswill, & Lurie-Beck, 2011).

Compensatory strategies addresses the regulation of loss as a function of aging or disability (Riediger, Li, & Lindenberger, 2006; Lindenberger, Lövdén, Michael Schellenbach, Li, & Krüger, 2008). It involves efforts (consciously or unconsciously) to maintain a given level of functioning despite decline in, or loss of, previously available resources (Riediger, Li, & Lindenberger, 2006; Lindenberger, Lövdén, Michael Schellenbach, Li, & Krüger, 2008;

Donorfio, Mohyde, Coughlin, & D'Ambrosio, 2008; Haustein et al., 2013; Monterde-i-Bort, 2004). Compensation, in contrast to optimization, aims at counteracting or avoiding losses rather than achieving higher levels of functioning (Riediger, Li, & Lindenberger, 2006). When driving, compensatory strategies could be a way to maintain the level of risk as described in the driver behavior models.

Older drivers often show a more defensive driving style with lower average speeds (Chipman, MacGregor, Smiley, & Lee-Gosselin, 1992; Haustein et al., 2013) and keep a larger following distance (Rajalin, Hassel, & Summala, 1997). Age-related changes in driving patterns can be seen as a strategy to compensate for age-related decline and thus prolong the period of independent safe mobility (Donorfio et al., 2008).

In psychology, coping refers to the use of conscious effort to solve personal and interpersonal problems, seeking to master, minimize or tolerate stress or conflict (e.g., Ben-Zur, 2009; Carver & Connor-Smith, 2010). One way of coping can be to simply avoid situations that cause stress or discomfort. Older drivers have been found to choose not to drive in certain conditions or environments and avoid risk-taking (Haustein et al., 2013). Driving conditions avoided by older drivers include rush hours, darkness, poor weather or road surface conditions, driving in unfamiliar areas (D'Ambrosio et al., 2008; Gwyther & Holland, 2012; Hakamies-Blomqvist, 1994; Rothe, 1990). Moreover, older drivers are less likely than middle-aged drivers to be engaged in distracting activities such as adjusting in-vehicle equipment or using a mobile phone (Fofanova & Vollrath, 2012; McEvoy, Stevenson, & Woodward, 2006). Avoidance of distracting activities while driving is one coping strategy.

To summarize, the ability to drive is affected by the deficits that come with age and lead to changes in driving behaviors. The behavioral patterns of older drivers are more cautious and include both compensatory strategies (e.g., lower speed, longer distance) and coping strategies (e.g., avoidance of certain situations or distracting activities).

Assessment of Driver Behavior

According to de Waard (1996), good reflectors of primary-task performance at the control level (c.f. Michon, 1985) are measures of lateral position (LP) and steering wheel (SW) movements and at the maneuvering level (c.f. Michon, 1985) include the time-to-line-crossing (TLC; Godthelp, 1984). Standard Deviation Lateral Position (SDLP) has been shown to be a sensitive performance measure (e.g., Hicks & Wierwille, 1979, O'Hanlon et al., 1982, O'Hanlon, 1984). De Waard (1996) showed that increased road complexity could lead to an increase in the SD of the SW movements, while the addition of a secondary task reduced the SD of the SW movements. Manipulation of both driving speed (e.g., Fuller, 2008; Summala, 2007; Levis-Evans, 2012) and degree of engagement in secondary tasks (Fuller, 2005) may be most important in maintaining the preferred level of risk.

Visual-search strategy has been shown to be indicative of informational needs (Hughes & Cole, 1988). According to de Waard (1996), eye-tracking measures are related to primary-task performance; however, they can also be used as a secondary-task performance measure in the case of embedded tasks. This is how eye tracking was used in the experimental studies in the present thesis. In the simulator study, driving was the primary task and an additional device was used for the secondary task. In the field study, drivers had to look at the navigation display to know which way to go. Relationships between frequency of fixation and instrument importance, as well as between length of fixations and difficulty in obtaining information from instruments, have been shown by Wilson and Eggemeier (1991). O'Donnell and Eggemeier (1986) reported that an increase in workload was accompanied by an increased fixation time.

Advanced Driver Assistance Systems

One approach to accident prevention and injury reduction is the introduction of in-vehicle-based preventive safety functions, also known as Advanced Driver Assistance Systems (ADAS) (e.g., lane-keeping support, adaptive cruise controllers, collision warning systems). In contrast to protective, or passive, in-vehicle safety functions (e.g., seat belt, airbag), whose purpose is to mitigate crash consequences, the general goal of ADAS is to prevent crashes from occurring at all. This is meant to be achieved either by alerting the driver to potential hazards (warning) or by taking over the driving task to some extent (intervention), using, for example, autonomous braking in emergency situations (Ljung Aust, 2012). Carsten and Nilsson (2001) made the distinction between information systems, that interact with the driver, and other intervening systems, that interact directly with the vehicle. Navigation systems are typical of the former category and adaptive cruise control of the latter.

An ADAS typically consists of one or more environment sensors mounted on the vehicle, for example radars or cameras. Software that uses sensor input determines what actions the ADAS should take and the particular driver or vehicle interface is used to alert the driver or control the vehicle. Examples of safety technologies, which fall under the ADAS umbrella, are Forward Collision Warning (FCW), Adaptive Cruise Control, Lane Departure Warning, and Drowsiness Warning (Ljung Aust, 2012).

A key issue for ADAS systems is to verify that they actually improve traffic safety. While the safety potential of ADAS can be affected by many factors, Carsten and Nilsson (2001) proposed that all safety implications can be classified as belonging to either of three general aspects: the function safety aspect (technical reliability of the system); the Human Machine Interaction (HMI) aspect (operating, and communicating with, the system); and the traffic safety aspect (system influence on driving behavior, including changes in interactions with other road users).

Relevant for both the HMI aspect and the traffic safety aspect is the multiple resource theory (MRT) presented by Wickens and Hollands (1999). This theory describes information processing with stages (perception, WM and cognition, responding), modalities (visual, auditory) and codes (verbal, spatial). An important implication of the difference between processing codes is the ability to judge which control to use for response. Manual control may reduce performance if there are heavy demands on spatial working memory, for instance while driving, whereas voice control may disturb the performance of tasks with heavy verbal demands (Wickens & Hollands, 1999).

The HMI aspect is central to the effect of HL on the use of driver assistance systems, since communication with the system must be set such that NH is not crucial, meaning that output cannot be only auditory. Several studies have shown that tactile support is an intuitive and effective way of presenting direction information and alerting drivers to potential collisions (van Erp & van Veen, 2004; Ho, Tan, & Spence, 2005; Ho, Reed, & Spence, 2006).

From the traffic safety aspect, this may release other heavily loaded sensory channels and therefore potentially provide a major safety enhancement.

Another issue is whether there are effects of HL on driving behavior. Concerning the fact that most HL is age-related, Li and Perkins (2007) showed that seniors view technology in the same way as the general public, and that education has a larger influence on the willingness to learn about new technology than age does. For training, simulators can be used to provide hands-on experience of new driver support systems and may therefore be valuable supportive tools for the elderly driver (Peters & Nielsen, 2007).

In sum, ADAS aim to increase traffic safety by preventing crashes. To make the systems accessible for drivers with HL, alternatives to auditory signals are necessary. Tactile signals have been shown to be effective and intuitive in warning and providing directional information.

General Aim and Research Questions

The general aim of this thesis is to investigate traffic safety and mobility for individuals with HL from a perspective of cognitive psychology by using subjective and objective performance indicators. With the limited previous research and knowledge on this specific topic, the approach has been necessary exploratory. Three studies were conducted: a questionnaire survey and two experimental studies, whereof one driving simulator study and one field study. The overall aim of the questionnaire study was to evaluate whether there were any differences related to HL with regard to the choice of transportation or on the view of hearing in transport situations. With the limited previous knowledge in the field, there were no expected differences between the groups. The studies following the questionnaire study had more specific research questions and expectations. Henceforth, the population included in the studies was older adults, in order to create homogenous groups and also because the majority of HL is age-related.

Based on the results from the survey, the driving simulator study was conducted to examine if HL had an effect on driving behavior or on increased workload. Gaze data was analyzed to compare visual behavior and in addition, the efficiency of a tactile signal to alert the driver was evaluated. A more cautious driving behavior was expected among the drivers with HL, because of compensatory strategies such as longer distance to other vehicles, lower driving speed and a more active visual search behavior. Coping strategies such as paying less attention to the secondary task were also expected.

A field study was conducted to replicate and validate the effects from the simulator study in real traffic. In the field study, the aim was to also evaluate a driver assistance system (navigation system) with a supportive tactile signal. Compensatory strategies such as slower driving speed and more glances in the mirrors were expected for the drivers with HL. The tactile support was expected to lead to more focus on the road, better driving performance and higher satisfaction with the system.

Methods

Ethical Considerations

In the studies presented in this thesis, the aim was to create as homogenous groups as possible with regard to age-related HL, and to control for vision loss and cognitive decline. Ethical considerations mainly concerned integrity issues (no data could be tracked back to any individual). Potential ethical problems identified in the studies include missing or lacking information with regard to the aim of the studies, the optional participation (participants could resign at any time without having to give any motive), the noncompulsory sharing of personal audiograms, and the receipt and treatment of the audiograms. All of the studies presented in this thesis were conducted during 2011-12 in Linköping and received ethical approval from the Research Ethics committee (Etikprövningsnämnden, EPN 2011/125-31; 2012/345-31) in Linköping.

Methodological Challenges

There were three different assessments to evaluate the effect of HL on traffic safety and mobility: the assessment of HL; the assessment of cognition, and the assessment of traffic safety each challenging and each with several possible methods. The results from each assessment were then to be put in relation to the other 2, which was even more challenging. Some of these challenges are presented in this section.

HL Population and Recruitment of Participants

Individuals with HL constitute a heterogeneous population due to a large variation in age, level of HL, and onset and cause of HL. Additionally, HL may be either unilateral or bilateral. This heterogeneity, in combination with the low level of knowledge in the area of HL and traffic safety, makes designs with sharp hypothesis-testing difficult to conduct. However, the population is large and thus, for the experimental studies and from a heterogeneous population included in the questionnaire study, we recruited as homogenous a group as possible. This was sensible and realistic, and provided a perspective based on the reality of those living with HL.

Geographical differences and variations in driving experience had also to be considered. Traffic situations may be very different in large cities and small towns, and individual driving experience may affect how people cope with any particular situation. However, in the studies included in this thesis, all participants were recruited from the same region and at least mileage per year and years with a driver's license was controlled for.

As well as HL, loss of vision is also a part of normal aging (e.g., Risacher et al., 2013; Heyl & Wahl, 2012). Wearing glasses can cause problems with eye tracking (Eachus, Cassidy, Norgate, Marrow, & Greene, 2008; O'Brien & Sharon, 2009), and this consideration restricted our potential participants. Furthermore, there will always be uncertainty of the representativeness of participants in any study. Not all individuals are willing to take part in research studies, and there is a risk that whatever characterizes those willing to participate from those not willing will lead to systematic sampling errors.

Response rate and completeness of questionnaires are difficult to control when participation is voluntary. There are arguments for and against using Internet (electronic) or paper and pencil versions. One advantage of electronic versions, besides the efficiency of receiving all answers in a database, is the opportunity to control that all questions have been answered before submission. However, paper versions have been found to have a higher response rate than electronic versions (73.2% compared to 17.9%, respectively) (Kongsved, Basnov, Holm-Christensen, & Hjollund, 2007).

Driving Simulator versus Real Driving

The advantages of performing simulator studies, including the opportunity to offer a safe convenient alternative to measuring driving performance on the road and the ability to keep driving conditions and environmental conditions constant, also come with limitations (Mullen, Charlton, Devlin, & Bédard, 2001; Nilsson, 1993). For example, motion, velocity and acceleration ranges are limited. It is impossible to fully represent a real traffic environment, and there is also the chance of simulator sickness, a type of motion sickness specifically experienced in simulators (Nilsson, 1993). Moreover, the simulated world does not contain the same level of detail and roughness as the real world. Since there is a limited amount of details in the simulated world, there is also less to focus on. It is not known how much this limitation affects visual behavior. Simulator performance shows medium to strong correlations with many on-road driving performance measures, and with other cognitive and physiological measures. However, simulators must be validated for each new setting (Mullen et al., 2001).

Challenges with Cognitive Assessments

One of the greatest concerns when creating a test for cognitive assessment is whether or not it actually measures what we think it is measuring. A test has construct validity if it demonstrates an association between the test scores and the prediction of a theoretical characteristic. Hughes, Sapp, and Kohler (2006) presented the challenges of conducting accurate cognitive assessments of students with HL. The authors pointed out that poor performance on an assessment may not necessarily indicate lower ability, but may be the result of a misunderstanding of the type or language of the assessment. Thus, they suggested using a variety of measures to assess participants, especially individuals with HL.

Procedures and Validity

Procedures and validity are first discussed for the questionnaire study and then for both of the experimental studies since several measures are included in the simulator study and the field study.

Questionnaire Study

Along with questions about hearing and transport habits, aspects found in the literature to be avoided by older drivers were included in the questionnaire (long distances, rush hours, darkness, poor weather, road surface conditions, and driving in unfamiliar areas) (D'Ambrosio, 2008; Gwyther, 2012; Hakamies-Blomqvist, 1994; Rothe, 1990). In the questions about traffic incidents and accidents definitions from a report from the Swedish Road Administration (STRADA, 2007) were used.

Questionnaire responses were mainly scored using a 5-point scale. The odd number was chosen to allow neutral answers, and 5 points was chosen instead of a larger number because the data were not expected to be skewed in either direction (Johnston, 2008). The alternatives of "*do not know*" or "*not relevant*" were also included to avoid forcing participants to tick wrong alternatives. A few open questions were also included to allow respondents to answer in their own words, and likewise after each closed question there was room for comments.

Experimental Studies

According to de Waard (1996), self-report scales and performance measures are the most appropriate for workload assessment, and a useful experimental design in traffic research is to compare task performance in an experimental (e.g., mental load) condition with performance under baseline conditions. Evaluation of workload due to complexity should, according to de Waard et al., either involve an increase in road complexity or an increase in task complexity, for example with the addition of a secondary task. This approach was used in both experimental studies. In the simulator study, load conditions with and without a secondary task were compared with baseline conditions with and without the secondary task. In the field study, road complexity varied between city and ring road, while task complexity either by varied including a tactile support in the navigation system or leaving that out. Self-report scales during (only in the simulator study) and after the drive were used, as well as performance measures.

Critical incidents, law violations, and LP errors are measures of driving performance and have been used as such in task-performance assessments (e.g., Pohlmann & Traenkle, 1994). In particular, complex behavior, such as the occurrence of critical incidents or behavior in a complex driving environment, can be easier, or more accurately, detected and judged by an observer than captured in a single performance measure (de Waard, 1996).

Pretests

In both experimental studies, hearing tests were performed on all drivers with NH and for participants with HL audiograms were provided from the audiology clinic. The inclusion criterion for the NH group was a hearing threshold of maximum 20 dB at each frequency (500, 1000, 2000, and 4000 Hz), measured with a pure tone audiometer. Inclusion criterion for the HL group was a moderate HL (41-60 dB) according to WHO categories (Arlinger, 2007), measured with a pure-tone average of 4 mean values, PTA4 (means of 500, 1000, 2000, and 4000 Hz). In the field study (Paper IV), more pretests were included to control for differences between the experimental groups. Apart from HL, normal consequences of aging also include declining visual abilities, such as visual acuity and contrast sensitivity (e.g., Risacher et al., 2013; Heyl & Wahl, 2012) and cognition (e.g., McDowd & Shaw, 2000; Verhaeghen et al., 2003; Mayr et al., 2001; Verhaeghen et al., 2005, Craik & Salthouse, 2000; Phillips & Lesperance, 2003). Relationships between sensory and cognitive losses in older adults have also been presented (Clay et al., 2009; Heyl & Wahl, 2012; Holland, 2009; Vreeken et al., 2013). Therefore, in the field study, vision tests and cognitive tests were included to control for differences between the groups. Clinical vision measures included binocular *distance visual acuity* using a logMAR chart (Ferris, Kassoff, Bresnick, & Bailey, 1982) and binocular *contrast sensitivity* (log CS) using the Pelli-Robson chart (Pelli, Robson,

& Wilkins, 1988). Cognitive tests included: *verbal ability* (The F-test, Psykologiförlaget, Stockholm); a cognitive test battery, including *physical matching*, *physical lexical matching*, *rhyme* and *reading span* (Hällgren, Larsby, Lyxell, & Arlinger, 2001); a computerized dynamic TMT, shown to be related to driving performance (Lehtonen, Dahlström, Hiltunen, & Summala, 2012), and the Useful Field of View test (UFOV), measuring skills thought to be used during driving (Ball & Owsley, 1993).

Secondary Task

In the simulator study, to create 2 levels of cognitive workload in the secondary task the phonological similarity effect was used (Conrad & Hull, 1964; Baddeley, 1968; Hitch & Halliday, 1983), and the sequences consisted of randomized letters that were either phonologically alike (e.g., BDPT) or not phonological alike (e.g., RKNJ). Each letter was displayed for 0.7 seconds, which is an adaptation of Sternberg's scanning paradigm (Sternberg, 1966). The display time had to be long enough for recognition of the letters, but short enough for the participants to keep their eyes on the display.

Performance Indicators

Performance indicators in the simulator study were mean LP, SDLP, minimum TLC (TLCmin; Brookhuis, Waard, & Fairclough, 2003), mean driving speed, SD driving speed, and secondary task performance. For subjective ratings during the simulator test drive, the following question was presented on the screen after each event: How critical did you experience the situation to be? The participants answered on a scale from 1 = not critical at all to 7 = extremely critical. This is an adaptation (specifically the dimension of the degree of complication) from the Situation Awareness Rating Technique (SART) 10 Dimension-scale, with each dimension ranging from 1-7 (Endsley & Garland, 2000). In the field study, mean driving speed and SD driving speed were included along with eye tracking (specifically frequency and length of fixations) and driving performance assessment according to an on-road protocol (Selander, Lee, Johansson, & Falkmer, 2011).

Table 1. Participants' demographic details and data collection method in the studies

Study	Participants	Gender (Male/Female)	Age Mean (SD) Male/Female	Data collection method
I	93 self-reported NH 48 mild HL 105 moderate HL 47 severe HL 18 profound HL	50/43 17/31 44/61 28/19 7/11	71.5 (13.2)/63.4 (14.5) 69.0 (11.1)/68.7 (12.4) 74.8 (7.7)/61.1 (15.9) 55.5 (15.1)/75.1 (14.7) 57.3 (12.6)/65.8 (9.7)	Questionnaire survey
II	24 NH 24 moderate HL	12/12 13/11	60.1 (7.1)/59.6 (5.0) 62.0 (7.9)/61.0 (9.8)	Driving simulator study with driving performance, eye tracking, and survey
III	16 NH 16 moderate HL	5/10 7/8	51.2 (8.3)/52.8 (11.0) 60.2 (12.4)/53.0 (13.3)	Field study with eye tracking, questionnaire and driving assessment

Participants and Data Collection

For the questionnaire survey, participants were recruited from the local branch of the Swedish hard of hearing association. A control group with normal hearing (NH), matched with age, gender and geographical location, was then selected from a commercial database. The survey was also used to recruit participants for the other studies by including a question about their interest in taking part in further research in the field of HL and traffic safety. The VTI participant database was used to recruit participants with NH. Information about participants' demographic details is listed in Table 1 together with the data collection method used for each study.

Design and Statistical Analyses

Questionnaire Survey

Logistic regression (binary for dichotomous questions answered by "yes" or "no" and ordinal for questions with more than 2 ordered alternatives) was used to analyze the results of the questionnaire study because it was explorative and had no inbuilt expectations to examine. This is a type of regression analysis with binary or ordinal response variables. The probabilities describing the possible outcomes of a single trial are modelled as a function of the explanatory (predictor) variables, using a logistic function (Bishop, 2006).

All predictor variables were entered simultaneously, since there was no presumption of which one would explain more. The results from the logistic regression are presented using odds ratio (*OR*), which quantifies how strongly the presence or absence of property A in the response variable is associated with the values on the predictor variables (McHugh, 2009; Mosteller, 1968). That is, this gives a measure of the influence of the predicting variables (e.g., degree of HL, gender, age) on the dependent variable (e.g., having a driver's license). $OR = 1$ means no influence, $OR > 1$ means an increasing probability, and $OR < 1$ means a decreasing probability.

Driving Simulator Study

The driving simulator study had a 2 × 2 × 2 factor design with the fixed factors *hearing status* (NH vs. HL), *gender* (men vs. women), and *difficulty level* (lower vs. higher). Participant (participants 1-48) within *hearing status* and *gender* was included as a random factor. On driving behavior measures (e.g., speed) and secondary task, analysis with planned comparisons within and between the Hearing status levels was carried out using a mixed model. For the post-trip questionnaire, with questions on subjects including subjective driving performance on ordinal scales, logistic regression and *OR* were used. Analysis of gaze data was conducted in 2 steps. The strategy for analyzing the distribution of glances was to start with a model as comprehensive as possible, with several variables, interactions, and multidimensional responses. A multivariate analysis of variance (MANOVA) was performed to examine whether *condition* (with or without secondary task), *hearing status*, *gender* or any two-factor interactions of these had an effect on the distribution of glances, where the distribution is governed by a vector representing the 7 target gaze zones. In this model, hearing, gender and condition were included as fixed variables, and a participant nested within hearing and gender was included as a random variable. The significant interaction effect of condition and hearing led to the analysis of each condition and each hearing status. ANOVA (analysis of variance) were performed to test hypotheses examining one zone at a time.

Field Study

In the field study a 2 × 2 × 2 factorial design with the between-groups factor *hearing status* (NH vs. HL), and the two within-groups factors *system information* (visual vs. visual tactile), and *complexity* (lower vs. higher) were used. Generalized estimating equations (GEEs) were used to model correlated data from this repeated measures design. GEEs are used to estimate the parameters of a generalized linear model with a possible unknown correlation between outcomes, and have the advantage of overcoming the classical assumptions of statistics, for example independence and normality, which are too restrictive for many problems (Liang & Zeger, 1986; James & Joseph, 2003).

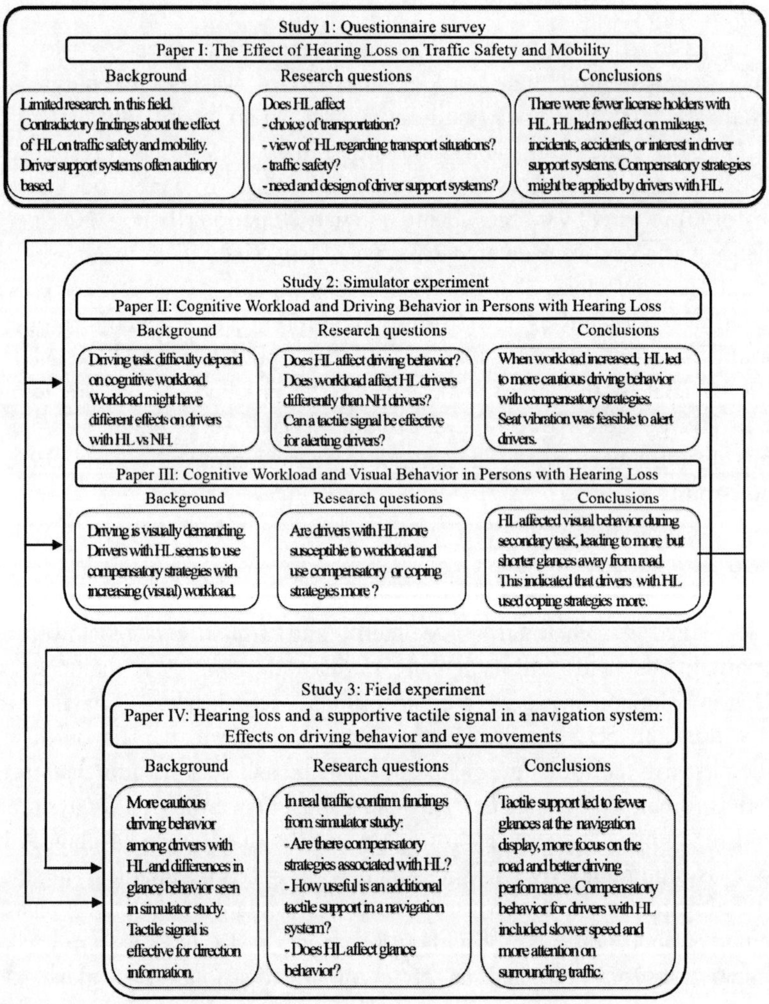

Figure 3. Overview of studies, papers and findings.

GEEs were used on the following linear or continuous outcome measures: speed, on-road performance, gaze behavior patterns, and usability questions. Predictor variables were *system information* (within subjects), *hearing category,* and *age* (between subjects). Outputs were Wald statistics (χ^2), showing the significance, and an unstandardized regression coefficient (*B*), presenting the relationship between the groups. For background questions in the questionnaire, cognitive tests, and vision tests one-way ANOVAs were performed.

Summary of Studies and Papers

In experimental psychology there are often several parts of a study presented in one paper. In this thesis, the studies are fewer and larger and have generated one or 2 papers each, which is more common in traffic safety research.

An overview of studies, papers, and findings is presented in Figure 2. Three studies were conducted and generated four scientific papers, which are included in this thesis. Since the initial level of knowledge was low and somewhat contradictory, a questionnaire study was the first step on the path to evaluate differences in traffic safety and mobility related to HL. The results from the first study are presented in the first scientific paper and also included in the background to the second study conducted in the driving simulator. The results from this study generated the second and third scientific papers and were (together with the results from the questionnaire study) included in the background to the third study conducted in real traffic. This study generated the fourth scientific paper. Summaries of each study are presented in the following sections.

Study 1: A Questionnaire Survey

Paper I: The Influence of Hearing Loss on Transport Safety and Mobility

Purpose

The purpose of study 1 was to examine how road users with different degrees of HL, compared to road users with NH, experience traffic safety and mobility. Specifically, three general research questions were investigated: how HL affects the choice of transportation type (e.g., driving your own car vs. public transport); personal view of HL in relation to transport situations, and the need for and design of driver support systems (e.g., collision warning, parking aid, navigation systems, lane keeping systems) for drivers with HL.

Method

A questionnaire survey was conducted with participants recruited from the local branch of the Swedish Association for Hard of Hearing People (HRF). A NH control group, random and matched by age, gender and geographical location, was selected from a commercial database. From audiogram data, participants were sorted into groups according to their degree of HL. A web-based questionnaire was constructed to capture the 3 research questions mentioned above. With assistance from HRF, letters were sent out to members of their local branches with an invitation to take part in the study. There was also the possibility of receiving a paper version of the questionnaire. The response rate was 35% (n = 194) in the group with HL and 42% (n = 125) in the group with NH. The individuals with hearing loss were grouped into four groups according to the degree of their hearing loss (mild, moderate, severe, and profound). After receiving permission from the participants, audiograms were provided by the local audiology clinic for the HL group.

Results

A higher degree of HL was associated with less likelihood of having a driver's license. However, individuals with HL who had a driver's license, drove as much as NH drivers. HL was related to the criteria for choosing the type of transport, such that individuals with more HL rated written information as more important and time cost and safety as less important than those with less HL. However, in the aggregate, no difference between the groups could be shown in the distribution of how much each mode of transportation was used.

With a few exceptions, HL did not affect the ratings of importance of hearing for different transportation types. The exceptions were walking and public transportation, where respondents with moderate HL rated hearing as significantly more important than those with NH. There was no effect of HL on involvement in incidents or accidents.

Degree of HL was related to several questions of driving ability, and the general pattern was that individuals with a higher degree of HL rated driving ability less affected by HL. This indicates that they might be using compensatory strategies. The interest in a warning system for inattention and the attitude toward strengthening of or complementing auditory information in traffic situations was high regardless of HL.

Conclusion

From this study, it was concluded that HL influences the prevalence of a driver's license and criteria for choosing type of transportation; however, HL has no effect on the distribution of how much each type of transportation was used. In general, respondents with more HL were less concerned about the effect of HL, indicating that they might be using compensatory strategies (adjustments to compensate for a decline). The interest in a warning system for inattention and the attitude toward strengthening of auditory information in traffic situations was high regardless of HL or not. This suggests a need for further research on compensatory strategies and on the design of support systems accessible for drivers with HL.

Study 2: A Driving Simulator Study

Purpose

A simulator study was conducted to compare the effect of cognitive workload in individuals with and without HL, respectively, in driving situations with varying degree of complexity. The effectiveness of a tactile signal used to call for driver attention was also evaluated.

Method

Twenty-four participants with moderate HL and 24 with NH experienced 3 different driving conditions: baseline driving on a 35-km long rural road with a speed limit of 70 km/hr; critical events with a need to act fast; and a parked car event with the possibility to adapt the workload to the situation (e.g., by deciding whether or not to focus on the secondary task). A secondary task (observation and recalling of 4 visually displayed letters) was present during the drive, with 2 levels of difficulty in terms of load on the phonological loop.

A tactile signal, presented by means of a vibration in the seat, was used to announce the secondary task and thereby simultaneously evaluated in terms of effectiveness when calling for driver attention. The letters were displayed on a screen at a low down angle, so that the driver had to look away from the road. Twice per minute, drivers were prompted by the tactile signal in the seat to first look at and then read back a complete sequence of 4 letters appearing on the display. The total duration of the task corresponds to a critical situation in which drivers take their eyes off the road to look at the display.

For the critical events, to create near collisions, the drivers were distracted by means of the secondary task, and then "pushed" across the median toward an oncoming vehicle by introducing a steering angle in the simulated vehicle without submitting this information to the motion platform. The parked car event was a situation when the participants saw a parked car ahead (from 360 meters) with warning lights activated. This study generated 2 papers with different focus presented separately below.

Paper II: Cognitive Workload and Driving Behavior in Persons with Hearing Loss

In this paper, objective driver behavior measures from the simulator study accompanied by subjective ratings during and after the test drive are presented, as well as the result from secondary task and the questionnaire after driving.

Method

Driver behavior measures were mean driving speed; SD of Driving speed; mean LP; SD of LP; and minimum time to line crossing. The secondary task was analyzed with respect to the number of correct recalled letters per task, number of skipped letters per task, and number of correct recalled letters per task ignoring the order. Subjective ratings during and after the test drive were included to evaluate the realism of the simulated event. There was also a questionnaire after driving including self-reported driving behavior, realism of the simulator, and evaluation of the tactile signal used to announce the secondary task.

Results

HL had no effect on driving behavior during baseline driving, where no events occurred. During both the secondary task and the parked car event, HL was associated with decreased mean driving speed compared with baseline driving. Participants with HL drove approximately 6 km/hr slower during the secondary task than NH participants did (approx. 65 km/hr vs. 70 km/hr), $F(1, 44) = 7.68$, $p = 0.01$, $\eta p2 = 0.14$. At the parked car event, participants with HL drove approximately 5 km/hr slower, $F(1, 44) = 2.42$, $p = 0.05$, $\eta p2 = 0.05$.

The effect of HL on the secondary task performance, both at baseline driving and at critical events, was more skipped letters and fewer correctly recalled letters. Furthermore, at critical events task difficulty affected participants with HL more. There was no effect of HL on the secondary task at the parked car event. Participants were generally positive about the use of a tactile signal in the seat as a means for announcing the secondary task. There was no effect of HL on self-reported driving performance.

Conclusion

It was concluded that differences in driving behavior and secondary task performance related to HL appear when demands increase, either when driving demands exceed baseline driving or when the secondary task becomes more cognitively demanding or both. Increased demands lead to a more cautious driving behavior with a decreased mean driving speed and less focus on the secondary task. This indicate that HL is associated with both compensatory strategies and coping strategies. Seat vibration was found to be a feasible way to alert drivers with or without HL.

Paper III: Cognitive Workload and Visual Behavior in Elderly Drivers with Hearing Loss

The objective of this paper was to compare visual behavior in individuals with NH and with moderate HL, and reveal possible differences by analyzing eye-tracking data from the simulator study.

Method

The cockpit was divided into 7 target zones: windshield, right, left, center mirror, speedometer, task display, other. Gaze data were analyzed with respect to distribution of glances, fixations in target zones and eye movement behavior. Eye gaze behavior was assessed during normal driving and driving with the loading secondary task. The following performance indicators were used: number of glances away from the road, mean duration of glances away from the road, maximum duration of glances away from the road, and the percentage of time when the driver was looking at the road. During the secondary task, additional eye movement data were assessed in terms of number of glances to the secondary task display, mean duration of glances to the secondary task display, and maximum duration of glances to the secondary task display.

Results

Vertical and horizontal gaze directions showed only small differences between the NH and HL groups, such that the HL group tended to have narrower and more distinct gaze manners corresponding to the speedometer and the mirrors in the cockpit. There were also some indications that, during the secondary task, the HL group looked in the center rear-view mirror and further to the right more often than the NH group. Also, it could be seen that glances toward the secondary task display were preceded by glances to the mirrors more often in the HL group than in the NH group.

The main result from the analysis of target zones (the objects that the driver looks at within the car's cockpit) was that during the secondary task, drivers with HL looked twice as often in the rear-view mirror as they did during normal driving and twice as often as drivers with NH regardless of the driving condition.

Also, during secondary task, drivers with HL showed a different strategy when looking away from road. They looked away from the road as much as drivers with NH; however, with more frequent glances of shorter duration.

Conclusion

It was concluded that differences in visual search behavior between drivers with NH and drivers with HL are bound to driving condition. During the secondary loading task, drivers with HL looked twice as often in the rear-view mirror than during normal driving and than drivers with NH, regardless of driving condition. Moreover, during secondary task, drivers with HL looked away from the road as much as drivers with NH, but with more frequent glances of shorter duration. The results also indicate that drivers with HL performed a visual scan of the surrounding traffic environment before looking away toward the secondary task display. This more active visual search behavior might indicate that drivers with HL use compensatory strategies to a higher extent than NH drivers.

Study 3: A Field Study in Real Traffic

Paper IV: Hearing Loss and a Supportive Tactile Signal in a Navigation System: Effects on Driving Behavior and Eye Movements

Purpose

The purpose of the third study, conducted in real traffic, was to replicate and further examine findings from previous simulator study, namely driver compensatory strategies associated with HL and evaluate possible effects of additional tactile support in a navigation system. Furthermore, since the simulator study indicated differences in gaze behavior between drivers with and without HL, eye-tracking data was analyzed as part of the study

Method

Thirty-two participants (16 HL and 16 NH) performed two pre-programmed navigation tasks in an urban environment. In one task, participants received only visual navigation information, while in the other vibration in the seat was used as a complement. This tactile support was given in the left or the right side of the driver's seat to indicate the direction of the next turn. Performance indicators and measures included driving speed, driving behavior observations (using a protocol filled out by a test leader), eye tracking, and a post-drive questionnaire. SMI glasses were used for eye tracking, recording the point of gaze within the scene. Analysis of gaze data was performed on predefined regions such as windscreen, mirrors, navigation display, and speedometer. The questionnaire examined participants' experience of the two navigation tasks in terms of their feelings of safety, usefulness, and comfort.

Results

On road sections with a speed limit of 70 km/hr, participants with a HL drove 4 km/hr slower than participants with NH. The same tendency was also seen on sections with a speed limit of 50 km/hr; however, this result was not statistically significant.

During observed driving, participants with NH had on average 0.3 more marks on the measure 'speed too high' than participants with HL, and participants with HL had 0.5 more marks on the measure 'speed too low' than those with NH. Participants with HL also averaged 1 mark higher on the measure 'uneven speed' than participants with NH.

Participants with HL spent on average 1.4% more time looking in the rear-view mirror than NH participants. HL participants looked an average of 3 times as often (0.3 times per minute vs. 0.1 times) in the rear-view mirror as the NH group, but there was no effect on the duration of glances.

When driving without the tactile information activated, participants had on average 0.5 more marks on the measure ‘inattention straight’ and 0.5 more marks on the measure ‘position distance’ than when they had the tactile information. With the tactile information activated, participants looked on average 7% less at the navigation display and consequently on average 7% more through the windscreen than without the tactile information. The number of glances per minute revealed that without the tactile information, on average participants looked once more per minute at the navigation display and there was no effect on the duration of glances. With the tactile information activated, both hearing groups were significantly more satisfied with their ability to navigate and with the help they got from the system. Participants also felt safer and more comfortable in this condition. Furthermore, participants in the HL group were significantly more satisfied than the NH group with their ability to navigate when the tactile information was activated. There was no effect of HL on self-rated driving performance.

Conclusion

Results from this study revealed that drivers with HL drove more slowly than drivers with NH, drove slower and looked more often in their rear-view mirror. These compensatory strategies suggest a more cautious driving behavior. The study also showed that tactile support leads to higher satisfaction with the navigation system, less time spent looking at the navigation display (in terms of frequency), and thus more focus on the road and better driving performance (in terms of both attention and distance).

General Discussion

The general aim of this thesis was to investigate traffic safety and mobility for older individuals with HL from the perspective of cognitive psychology. With the limited previous research and relatively low level of knowledge in this field the approach has been exploratory with subjective and objective performance indicators, and the findings from each study have been included for further evaluation.

The questionnaire survey investigated how HL affects the choice of transportation, personal views of HL in relation to transport situations, and the design requirements for driver support systems accessible for road users with HL. The simulator study examined differences in driving behavior and visual behavior between drivers with NH and drivers with HL and the effectiveness of a tactile signal to alert drivers. The field study further examined possible compensatory strategies associated with HL, the usefulness of an additional tactile support in a navigation system, and differences in eye movement patterns.

Summary of Results

Summarizing and abstracting the effects of HL throughout the studies included in this thesis reveal that the effects of HL on traffic safety and mobility are existing, but small (in terms of effect sizes), often bound to workload condition and rather specific, but still consistent in the replicated studies.

The questionnaire revealed that differences in transportation habits related to HL include the less likelihood of having a driver's license and a higher valuing of written information, with the latter possibly prioritized before time and safety issues. Moreover, respondents with more HL were less concerned about the effect of HL, indicating that they might be using compensatory strategies. In addition, the interest in a warning system and the attitude toward strengthening of or complementing auditory information in traffic situations was high regardless of hearing ability. These are all new findings, pointing to a few potentially important effects of HL from a traffic safety and mobility perspective.

Furthermore, the questionnaire revealed that HL was not related to the frequency of using any of the transportation types (e.g., cars, cycling, or public transportation). There was no difference in the patterns with regard to transportation types during wintertime or any effect of HL on self-reported incidents or accidents.

In the experimental studies, differences related to HL in terms of driving behavior (mostly lower driving speed) were bound to driving conditions and occurred when the complexity of driving task increased (simulator study) or at a higher speed limit (field study). There was also an effect of HL on visual behavior, indicated in the simulator study and confirmed in the field study. Drivers with HL had a more active visual behavior with more frequent glances on the secondary task (simulator study), more frequent glances in the rear-view mirror, and more general scanning of the environment before looking away from the road (simulator study). Secondary task performance was lower for the HL group, with more skipped letters, suggesting this group is less willing to perform this task. These are all new findings, in line with the expectations, and the effect of HL on driving behavior and on visual search behavior suggest people with HL use more compensatory strategies and coping strategies leading to a more cautious driving behavior.

The tactile signal in the driver seat was found useful in both experimental studies, both for driver attention and for facilitating navigation with a GPS navigation device. The field study showed that the tactile support led to higher satisfaction with the navigation system. The tactile support also led to less time spent looking at the navigation display, and thus more focus on the road and better driving performance in terms of both attention and distance. These are new findings, supporting the expectations and adding to the growing body of evidence of the benefits of using tactile information in cars (van Erp & van Veen, 2004; Ho, Tan, & Spence, 2005; Ho, Reed, & Spence, 2006).

In the simulator study (study II), HL had no effect on driving behavior at baseline driving, where no events occurred and when no secondary task was present. In the field study, the effect of HL on driving speed displayed the same pattern, however was not significantly lower, at the lower speed limit. In neither of the experimental studies, there was an effect of HL on the self-rated driving performance.

Choice of Transportation

ICF, conceptualizing functioning and disability as an interaction between an individual's health condition, contextual factors of the environment and personal factors, includes mobility in activity and participation (WHO, 2001). There were some effects of HL found, which according to the hierarchical model suggested by Michon (1985), belong to the top level, where strategic decisions are made by control processing such as the choice of type of transport.

That the likelihood of having a driver's license is negatively associated with the degree of HL is a new finding. There was no effect of HL on mileage and also no relation between the degree of HL and driving cessation. This suggests that in the studied population difficulties or lack of interest associated with HL and car driving emerge when deciding whether or not to learn to drive. This is an indication of individuals with HL using coping. Knowing that difficulty in taking part in activities increase with the degree of HL (Gopinath, Schneider, Hickson, et al., 2012a; Grue et al., 2009; Wallhagen et al., 2001; Schneider et al., 2010), one could speculate that taking driving lessons might be too difficult for some individuals with HL, as some respondents mentioned. The main focus in this thesis is on those with moderate HL who are still driving; however, this driver's license issue is something for further research, since car access can act as a compensational tool for functional limitations (Sirén & Hakamies-Blomqvist, 2004, 2009) and is associated with better health and well-being among the elderly (Ellaway, Macintyre, Hiscock, & Kearns, 2003; Macintyre, Hiscock, Kearns, & Ellaway).

That individuals with HL sometimes find written information more important than time cost, and safety issues is also a new finding. According to Rumar (1988), there is always a risk in being mobile, and risk can be divided into statistical and experienced risk. There is a possibility that individuals with HL feel safer when they have written information and therefore prioritize this before statistical safety and time cost. Furthermore, individuals with moderate HL expressed a higher need to be able to hear on public transportation than those with NH. This is in line with Gopinath et al. (2012), who found that using public transportation is harder for individuals with HL, and there might be a need for more written information on public transportation to increase experienced safety, activity and participation for individuals with HL.

Driving Behavior

Motivational driving behavior models all have in common maintenance of the acceptable level of risk (Wilde, 1982; Fuller & Santos, 2002; Fuller, 2005, 2007; Fuller et al., 2008; Fuller, McHugh et al., 2008; Vaa et al., 2000; Vaa, 2003, 2007, 2011; Näätänen & Summala, 1974). Consistent with results from Wu et al. (2014), effects on driving behavior for individuals with HL emerge when driving task exceeds baseline driving. The main effects from the simulator study are consistent with Fuller (2005), suggesting that manipulating driving speed and engagement in a secondary tasks are the primary mechanisms for maintaining the preferred level of difficulty.

Lewis-Evans (2012) concluded that speed is not only a conscious choice but rather a challenge to be handled, at least on some level, by automatic processes, and that the existence of these processes can be inferred when the cognitive capability of drivers is loaded. There is a higher risk of cognitive fatigue in individuals with HL, and also possibly a different perception of speed (cf. Evans, 1970; Ohta & Komatsu, 1991). Taking this together, there is a possibility that drivers with HL may have decreased speed control, and therefore drive slower and at a more uneven speed (field study).

In addition, considering Lewis-Evans' (2012) suggestion that there is a threshold to account for the perception of subjective variables (e.g., task difficulty, effort, comfort, crash risk, and feeling of risk), drivers with HL might experience an increased feeling of risk (Rumar, 1988) and therefore aim to maintain a different level of risk. This increased feeling of risk might come from a decreased perception of the surroundings and decreased feedback leading to a decreased feeling of control, which is also reflected in the gaze behavior. That is, they might compensate for the increased risk by driving at a lower speed (e.g. Haustein et al., 2013), and be less engaged in distracting activities, which is a coping strategy (e.g., Ben-Zur, 2009; Fofanova & Vollrath, 2012).

Visual Behavior

Drivers with HL showed more watchful manners with regard to visual behavior. The higher frequency of glances in the mirrors point to the fact that individuals with HL might value this kind of information more than that with NH. This new finding is in line with the expectations of a compensatory strategy with a more active visual search behavior, due to the fact that hearing gives us valuable spatial and temporal resolution. This is also in line with Wilson and Eggemeier (1991), who found a relationship between frequency of fixation and instrument importance, and this, might be a part of a compensatory behavior.

Visual search strategy is according to traffic inspectors the most important concept related to risk awareness (Lidestam et al., 2010). The difference between drivers with HL and drivers with NH in the strategy of looking away from the road was apparent during the secondary task in the driving simulator. Drivers with HL looked away more often and for a shorter period each time; however, there was no effect of HL on total time with the eyes off the road. Again, this behavior might be connected to the experienced safety and feeling of risk, suggesting that avoiding long glances away is a coping strategy on the part of those with HL.

With the descriptive and explorative approach of this thesis, the relationship between the secondary task performance in Paper II and the gaze behavior in Paper III is interesting. In Paper II, we concluded that drivers with HL might be less willing to make an effort to perform the secondary task. Their lower performance might also be due to the fact that the task loads on the phonological loop and is thus more cognitively demanding for drivers with HL. An acquired HL may lead to a deteriorated function in the phonological loop, which means that drivers with HL should need to look at the letters for a longer time. However, as seen in Paper III, on the contrary they look at the secondary task display more frequently and with shorter duration compared to drivers with NH. This indicates that with the limited capacity during the secondary task, which also results in decreased speed for drivers with HL, driving safety is prioritized before performance on the task, which could be a sign of compensatory behavior.

Driver Assistance Systems

In the questionnaire survey, the interest in driver assistance systems was not affected by HL and suggested evaluation of alternative modality for driver support systems. From the classifications suggested by Carsten and Nilsson (2001), the HMI aspect (operating and communicating with the system) and the traffic safety aspect (system influence on driving behavior, including changes in interactions with other road users) are relevant for evaluating the effect of HL. Concerning the HMI aspect, and in line with the expectations and previous findings (e.g. van Erp & van Veen, 2004;), the tactile signal in the driver's seat was useful in both experimental studies, for both calling for driver attention and facilitating navigation with a GPS device. Furthermore, of high relevance for the traffic safety aspect, regardless of hearing status, the tactile support led to higher satisfaction with the navigation system, less time spent looking at the navigation display, more focus on the road, and better driving performance. This was in line with the expectations too, and may increase traffic safety for drivers regardless of HL or not, since this may release other heavily loaded sensory channels (c.f. Wickens and Hollands, 1999) and therefore potentially provide a major safety enhancement.

Methodological Discussion

The advantages of performing a simulator study also come with limitations (Mullen, Charlton, Devlin, & Bédard, 2001; Nilsson, 1993). For example, motion, velocity and acceleration ranges are limited, it is impossible to fully represent a real traffic environment, and participants may suffer from simulator sickness, a type of motion sickness experienced only in simulators (Nilsson, 1993).

There was an effect of HL, such that drivers with NH experienced the simulator as more realistic. Also, some effects of eye movement behavior indicated in the simulator were confirmed in the field study. These two effects might be related, such that the realism was needed for some of the effects to show. Also, female drivers with HL reported the highest values of simulator sickness, which might be connected to the realism of the simulator, such that higher experienced realism lead to less simulator sickness.

Age-related HL is the most common type of HL and thus it is most relevant to look at the effects of HL in the group of older people. With a quasi-experimental design (HL vs. NH) follows a heterogeneity between groups. To create as homogenous groups as possible, apart from hearing status, the aim was to recruit participants under 65 years of age to avoid age effects.

Conclusion

From the studies included in this thesis, it can be concluded that there are effects of HL on both traffic safety and mobility, such that individuals with HL are less likely to have a driver's license, more likely to show a more cautious driving behavior, and will sometimes prioritize experienced safety before statistical safety. The effects of HL revealed in this thesis are new findings and add to the knowledge and understanding of the influence of HL on traffic safety and mobility. Differences found consistently point to a generally more cautious behavior, which suggests an effect of HL on experienced safety.

Compensatory strategies and coping strategies associated with HL are bound to driving complexity and appear when complexity increases. These strategies include driving at lower speeds, using a more comprehensive visual search behavior (compensatory) and being less engaged in distracting activities (coping).

The influence of HL on the choice to drive a car is limited to the decision of whether or not to learn to drive, since HL does not affect mileage or driving cessation.

Evaluation of a tactile signal suggests that by adding a tactile modality, some driver assistance systems can also be made accessible to drivers with HL. At the same time, the systems might be more effective for all users, since visual resources can be more focused on the road, which could generally increase both traffic safety and mobility.

Based on the results in this thesis, drivers with HL cannot be considered an increased traffic safety risk, and there should be no need for adjustments of the requirements of hearing for a license to drive a car.

Suggestions for Future Research

This thesis presents exploratory and experimental research on the effects of HL on traffic safety and mobility. Some effects of HL have been found (suggesting a more cautious driving behavior), which can be used in future recommendations. There are also some aspects worth looking into further. Generally, it is possible that individuals with disabilities (of different kinds) might contribute to a better understanding of how to design better driver support systems. Since they are more sensitive to higher workload, they might be able to indicate how to develop support systems, which might be more useful for all drivers.

The compensatory strategies found, indicating maintenance of a different level of difficulty, suggest further investigation of the effect of HL on feeling of risk.

The possibility of individuals with HL experiencing higher safety when there is written information and therefore prioritizing this before statistical safety and time cost is worth further evaluation.

The accessibility of written information on public transportation is relevant to evaluate, since differences appeared in this and other studies (Gopinath et al., 2012b) related to the degree of HL.

Less likelihood of having a driver's license suggests further evaluation of the driving lesson situation for individuals with HL.

Positive effects of tactile signals in driver assistance systems suggest further research on how to implement accessible signals in these systems.

The effect of the use of hearing aid technologies when driving should be further investigated. This was not included in the studies presented in this thesis although there is reason to believe that the right aid can increase traffic safety and mobility (e.g., McCloskey, Koepsell, Wolf, & Buchner, 1994; Wu et al., 2014).

The fact that there is a decline in various abilities (e.g., cognitive, visual, auditory) associated with normal aging, makes further examination of the effects of decline in each type and combination of types, and also the effects of aid for each type, relevant for future study.

The effects of HL on perception and decision-making have not been examined explicitly in studies presented in this thesis. However, the results pointing at a difference in experienced safety associated with HL suggest that these aspects should be further studied.

The studies included in this thesis focus on age-related HL. It would be of interest to look at the effects of other types of HL such as genetic deafness or individuals with CI.

It would be relevant to study the effects of HL on cognitive fatigue and of cognitive fatigue on traffic safety, since cognitive fatigue is a known effect of HL (e.g. Moradi et al., 2014; Rönnberg et al., 2013) and could lead to decreased attention. Also, studying the effect of reducing cognitive fatigue on traffic safety can add to the understanding of the problem.

In this field of research, investigation into specific effects of decline in different aspects of EF, rather than attention to the broad perspective, is more likely to yield a more comprehensive picture.

It could be worthwhile to study other modalities of driver assistance systems than auditory and tactile, such as ambient (light), and to evaluate which modalities and ways of presenting the information are most suitable to which driver group or in which situations.

Acknowledgments

Many people contributed to this work in many different ways and made the PhD journey possible, more solid, or simply more enjoyable. I want to express my greatest thanks to:

All the wonderful participants, who took part in my studies, shared your ideas, and showed your great interest in my work.

My boss *Jan Andersson*, the coaching master, for making this possible. You liked this idea from the start and you have supported me all the way with your positive attitude and enthusiasm.

Björn Lyxell, my main supervisor. Your professional way of restricting the study population and guiding me towards sensible frames was invaluable, as were your friendly phone calls just to check on how things were going. I also appreciate how you led me through the funding jungle, resulting in 4 great months in Australia for me and my family.

Björn Peters, who was concerned that co-supervising me would affect our friendship. Well, I was not concerned at all, and I believe I was right. You showed great generosity in inviting me to and inspiring me in your area of expertise, which is one of the main reasons I enjoy working with you. I am also grateful for your establishment of national and international contacts for me.

Björn Lidestam, my co-supervisor. Although you often expressed doubts about your own contribution to this work, I have always appreciated your involvement. You have the ability to recognize the most essential and most interesting results and a remarkable way of un-complicating things by breaking them down to pieces. I look forward to working more with you now that you have joined our group.

Louise Hickson, for your positive response to my query on visiting you as a guest PhD student. Thanks to you, *Joanne Wood*, *Alex Black,* and *Alicja Malicka*, my time at QUT and

UQ in Brisbane was both enlightening and enjoyable. I look forward to future collaborations between our groups.

I am fortunate to work at an institute where people are professional, friendly, and truly helpful. *Lena Nilsson*, you are the one who first hired me and recommended me to the ergonomics course, and this was crucial in the decisions that led me to where I am now. *Jonas Jansson*, you handed over a simulator project to me at a perfect time and this allowed me to collect a great amount of data in a short time, resulting in 2 published papers. *Christer Ahlström*, co-writer and dedicated data analyst, I appreciate your efficient and exemplary way of working, whether with study planning, data processing, or writing. *Olle Eriksson*, co-writer and statistics expert, I am grateful for your never-ending patience with my statistics questions and your good collaboration on Paper III. Thanks are also due to many colleagues, who with their expertise have all contributed in some valuable way to the studies: *Anders Andersson, Jonas Andersson Hultgren, Björn Blissing, Anne Bolling, Anders Genell, Per Henriksson, Kristina Kindgren, Lena Levin, Katarina Nestor, Beatrice Söderström, Gunilla Sörensen, Harry Sörensen.*

During my years at VTI, I have met some of my best friends. *Sara Nygårdhs*, thank you for simply being the genuine you. *Katja Kircher*, regardless of how busy you are, you always find the time to stay updated on and support my activities. *Magnus Hjälmdahl*, *Jessica Berg*, and *Therese Jomander*, the chats we have during lunch, coffee breaks, and between breaks are invaluable and the first thing I miss when I am away. *Jerker Sundström,* thank you for this advice: If you ever go for a PhD, chose a subject that really interests you. *Malin Eliasson*, I have always appreciated your rationality and never-ending energy.

I am grateful for the colleagues that I got to know at the Disability Research Division and HEAD graduate school. Specifically, I want to thank *Håkan Hua*, for being a good friend through this journey and also for sharing your knowledge on Audiology; *Jakob Dahl*, for our interesting discussions on any topic; *Claes Möller*, for good and recurring email discussions on balance and motion sickness; *Shahram Moradi* for sharing your knowledge on cognitive fatigue; *Malin Wass*, for sharing your experience on how to apply for grants and go to Australia; *Mary Rudner*, for your guidance through the special research project, definitely my best course, and *Maria Hugo Lindén* for your fine administrative help, including organizing ticket and room bookings for courses located in other cities.

I have met many helpful people here and there to whom I want to express my thanks: *Birgitta Larsby* for lending me equipment, sharing your knowledge on audiology and helping me with participant recruitment. I am looking forward to more collaborations with you!; *Therese Bohn Eriksson* and *Henrik Lindgren* and the audiology clinics in Linköping and Norrköping for providing audiograms on the recruited participants; *HRF,* and in particular *Jan-Olof Bergold*, *Diego Hedman*, and *Lautaro Aranda,* for your cooperation with participant recruitment and input on the questionnaire; *Kenneth Holmqvist* for lending me the eye-tracking equipment, sharing your knowledge, and cooperating so helpfully in the field study, *Nicholas Herbert* for good teamwork in the field study. I hope we get a chance to work together again in the future, and the father of WM, *Alan Baddeley*, for responding so quickly and helpfully to my email with a question about display time.

A big thank to my near and dear ones, my family and friends, for being my source of energy. You all know who you are and that I love to have you around! Among these, a special thanks to *Mum* and *Dad*, for always believing in me, and being constantly supportive but never intrusive, and to my cousin *Mattias*, for your great interest in what I am doing and your instant support in the English language.

Finally, my wise and loving husband *Tobias,* thank you for being just the way you are, my favorite person. I love you.

References

Andersson, U. (2002). Deterioration of the phonological processing skills in adults with an acquired severe hearing loss. *European Journal of Cognitive Psychology,* 14(3), 335-352.

Andersson, U., & Lyxell, B. (1999). Phonological deterioration in adults with an acquired severe hearing impairment. *Scandinavian Audiology,* 28(4), 241-247.

Andersson, U., Lyxell, B., Rönnberg, J. & Spens, K.-E. (2001). Cognitive correlates of visual speech understanding in hearing-impaired individuals. *Journal of Deaf Studies and Deaf Education,* 6, 103-116.

Arlinger, S. (2003). Negative consequences of uncorrected hearing loss – A review. *International Journal of Audiology,* 42(2), 17-20.

Arlinger, S. (Ed.) (2007). *Nordisk Lärobok i Audiologi* [Nordic textbook of audiology]. Bromma: C-A Tegnér AB.

Atkinson, R. C., & Shiffrin, R. M. (1968). *Human memory: A proposed system and its control processes.* In K. W. Spence & J. T. Spence (Eds), The psychology of learning and motivation (Vol 2). New York: Academic Press. pp. 89-195.

Ausmeel H. (1988). *TIPS (Text-Information-Processing-System): A user's guide.* Linköping, Sweden: Department of Education and Psychology, Linköping University.

Baddeley, A. (2012). Working memory: Theories, models, and controversies. *Annual Revue of Psychology* 63, 1-29.

Baddeley, A. D. (1968). How does acoustic similarity influence short term memory? *Quarterly Journal of Experimental Psychology,* 20, 249-264.

Baddely, A. (2000). The episodic buffer: a new component of working memory? *Trends in Cognitive Sciences,* 4(11), 417-423.

Baddeley, A. (1983). Working memory. *Philosophical Transactions of the Royal Society,* 302, 311–324.

Ball, K., & Owsley, C. (1993). The Useful Field of View Test: a new technique for evaluating age-related declines in visual function. *Journal of the American Optometric Association,* 64(1), 71-79.

Ball, K., Owsley, C., Sloane, M. E., Roenker, D. L., & Bruni, J. R. (1993). Visual-attention problems as a predictor of vehicle crashes in older drivers. *Investigative Ophthalmology & Visual Science,* 34(11), 3110-3123.

Ball, K., Owsley, C., Stalvey, B., Roenker, D. L., Sloane, M. E., & Graves, M. (1998). Driving avoidance and functional impairment in older drivers. *Accident Analysis & Prevention,* 30, 313-323.

Baltes, P. B. & Lindenberger, U. (1997). Emergence of a powerful connection between sensory and cognitive functions across the adult life span: a new window to the study of cognitive aging? *Psychology and Aging,* 12, 12-21.

Banister, D., & Bowling, A. (2004). Quality of life for the elderly: the transport dimension. *Transport Policy,* 11(2), 105-115.

Ben-Zur, H. (2009). Coping styles and affect. *International Journal of Stress Management,* 16(2), 87-101.

Bishop, C. M. (2006). *Pattern recognition and machine kearning.* New York: Springer-Verlag.

Bonnel, W. (1999). Giving up the car: older women's losses and experiences. *Journal of Psychosocial Nursing and Mental Health Services,* 37, 10-15.

Bopp, K. L., & Verhaeghen, P. (2005). Aging and verbal memory span: a meta-analysis. *Journals of Gerontology Series B: Psychological Sciences and Social Sciences,* 60(5), 223-233.

Bowles, R. P., & Salthouse, T. A. (2008). Vocabulary test format and differential relations to age. *Psychology and Aging,* 23(2), 366-376.

Brayne, C., Dufouil, C., Ahmed, A., Dening, T. R., Chi, L-Y., McGee, M., & Huppert, F. A. (2000). Very old drivers: Findings from a population cohort of people aged 84 and over. *International Journal of Epidemiology,* 29(4), 704-707.

Brookhuis, K. A., Waard, D. D., & Fairclough, S. H. (2003). Criteria for driver impairment. *Ergonomics,* 46(5), 443-445.

Brickman A. M., & Stern Y. (2009). *Aging and memory in humans.* In: L.R. Squire (Ed.) Encyclopedia of Neuroscience (Vol. 1) Oxford: Academic Press. pp. 175-180.

Carsten, O., & Nilsson, L. (2001). Safety assessment of driver assistance systems. *European Journal of Transport and Infrastructure Research,* 1(3), 225-243.

Carver, C. S., & Connor-Smith, J. (2010). "Personality and Coping". *Annual Review of Psychology,* 61, 679-704.

Catchpole, K., & McKeown, D. (2007). A framework for the design of ambulance sirens. *Ergonomics,* 50(8), 1287-1301.

Cerella, J. (1990). *Aging and information-processing rate.* In: J.E. Birren, & K.W. Schaie (Eds.), Handbook of the psychology of aging, 3rd ed. San Diego, CA: Academic Press, pp. 201-221.

Charlton, J. L., Oxley, J., Fildes, B., Oxley, P., & Newstead S. (2003). Self-regulatory behaviours of older drivers. *Annual Proceedings Advancement of Automotive Medicine,* 47, 181-194.

Chipman, M. L., MacGregor, C. G., Smiley, A. M., & Lee-Gosselin, M. (1992). Time vs. distance as measures of exposure on driving surveys. *Accident Analysis & Prevention,* 24(6), 679-684.

Classon, L. (2013) *Phonological decline and compensatory working memory in acquired hearing impairment.* Doctoral Dissertation. The Swedish Institute for Disability Research. Linköping University.

Clay, O. J., Edwards, J. D., Ross, A. L., Okonkwo, O., Wadley, V. G., Roth, D. L., & Ball, K. K. (2010). Visual function and cognitive speed of processing mediate age-related decline in memory span and fluid intelligence. *Journal of Aging Health,* 21(4): 547-566.

Conrad, R., & Hull, A. J. (1964). Information, acoustic confusion and memory span. *British Journal of Psychology,* 55, 429-437.

Conway A. R., Kane M. J., & Engle R. W. (2003). Working memory capacity and its relation to general intelligence. *Trends in Cognitive Sciences,* 7(12): 547-552.

Craik, F. I. M., & Salthouse, T. A. (2000). *The handbook of aging and cognition* (Second ed.). London: Lawrence Erlbaum Associates.

D'Ambrosio, L. A., Donorfio, L. K. M., Coughlin, J. F., Mohyde, M., & Meyer, J. (2008). Gender differences in self-regulation patterns and attitudes toward driving among older adults. *Journal of Women & Aging,* 20(3-4), 265-282.

Daneman, M. & Carpenter, P. (1980). Individual differences in working memory and reading. *Journal of Verbal Learning and Verbal Behavior,* 19, 450-466.

Daneman, M. & Merikle, P. M. (1996). Working memory and language comprehension: a meta-analysis. *Psychonomic Bulletin and Review,* 3, 422-433.

De Lorenzo, R. A., & Eilers, M. A. (1991). A review of emergency warning systems. *Annals of Emergency Medicine,* 20(12), 1331-1335

De Waard, D. (1996). *The measurement of drivers' mental workload.* Thesis. University of Groningen, Netherlands.

Dellinger, A. M., Kresnow, M., White, D. D., & Sehgal, M. (2004). Risk to self versus risk to others: how do older drivers compare to others on the road? *American Journal of Preventive Medicine,* 26(3), 217-221.

Diamond, A. (2013). Executive functions. *Annual Review of Psychology,* 64, 135-168.

Dillén, J., Schmidt, L., & Jarlebring, I. (2005). *Äldre personers resvanor och aktiviteter* [Older adults' travel habits and activities]. Solna: Transek.

Dimitrijevic, A., John, M. S., & Picton, T. W. (2004). Auditory steady-state responses and word recognition scores in normal-hearing and hearing-impaired adults. *Ear and Hearing*, 25, 68-84.

Donorfio, L. K. M., Mohyde, M., Coughlin, J., & D'Ambrosio, L. (2008). A qualitative exploration of self-regulation behaviors among older drivers. *Journal of Aging & Social Policy,* 20(3), 323-339.

Eachus, P., Cassidy, S., Norgate, S., Marrow, L., & Greene, L. (2008). *Internet self-efficacy and visual search strategies: The use of eye tracking technology in the development of web-based learning resources.* Informing Science & IT Education Conference. Varna, Bulgaria.

Edwards, J. D., Lunsman, M., Perkins, M., Rebok, G. W., & Roth D. L (2009). Driving cessation and health trajectories in older adults. *Journals of Gerontology Series A: Biological Sciences and Medical Sciences,* 64(12), 1290-1295.

Ferris, F. L., Kassoff, A., Bresnick, G. H., & Bailey, I. (1982). New visual acuity charts for clinical research. *American Journal of Ophthalmology,* 94, 91-96.

Ellaway, A., Macintyre, S., Hiscock, R., & Kearns, A. (2003). In the driving seat: psychosocial benefits from private motor vehicle transport compared to public transport. *Transportation Research Part F: Traffic Psychology and Behaviour,* 6, 217-231.

Elliott, E. M., Cherry, K. E., Brown, J. S., Smitherman, E. A., Jazwinski, S. M., Yu, Q., & Volaufova, J. (2011). Working memory in the oldest-old: evidence from output serial position curves. *Memory & Cognition,* 39(8), 1423-1434.

Endsley, M. R., & Garland, D. J. (2000). *Situation awareness analysis and measurement.* London: Lawrence Erlbaum Associates.

Engle, R. W., Tuholski, S. W., Laughlin, J. E., Conway, A. R. (1999). Working memory, short-term memory, and general fluid intelligence: A latent-variable approach. *Journal of Experimental Psychology: General* 128(3), 309-31.

Englund, L. (Ed.). (2001). *Medicinska förhållanden av betydelse för innehav av körkort - Hörsel och balanssinne* [Medical conditions of importance for obtaining a driving license]: Vägverket, Trafikmedicinska rådet.

Evans, L. (1970). Speed estimation from a moving automobile. *Ergonomics,* 13(2).

Eysenck, M. W., & Keane, M. T. (2010). *Cognitive psychology: a student's handbook* (6th ed.): East Sussex: Psychology Press.

Farquhar, M. (1995). Elderly people's definitions of quality of life. *Social Science & Medicine,* 41(10), 1439-1446.

Fitzgibbons, P. J., & Gordon-Salant, S. (2010). *Behavioral studies with aging humans: Hearing sensitivity and psychoacoustics* In S. Gordon-Salant, R. D. Frisina, A. Popper, & D. Fay (Eds.), The aging auditory system: Perceptual characterization and neural bases for presbyacusis. Berlin: Springer.

Fofanova, J., & Vollrath, M. (2012). Distraction in older drivers –a face-to-face interview study. *Safety Science,* 50(3), 502-509.

Fonda, S. J., Wallace, R. B., & Herzog, A. R. (2001). Changes in driving patterns and worsening depressive symptoms among older adults. *Journals of Gerontology Series B: Psychological Sciences and Social Sciences,* 56B (6), 343-351.

Forrest, K. Y. Z., Bunker, C. H., Songer, T. J., Cohen, J. H., & Cauley, J. A. (1997). Driving patterns and medical conditions in older women. *Journal of the American Geriatrics Society,* 45(10), 1214-1218.

Frisina, D. R., & Frisina, R. D. (1997). Speech recognition in noise and presbycusis: relations to possible neural mechanisms. *Hearing Research,* 106(1-2), 95-104.

Fuller, R. (2000). The Task Capability Interface Model of the driving process. *Recherche Transports Sécurité*, 66, 47-59.

Fuller, R. (2005). Towards a general theory of driver behaviour. *Accident Analysis & Prevention,* 37(3), 461-472.

Fuller, R. (2007). *Motivational determinants of control in the driving task.* In: P. Cacciabue (Ed.), Modelling driver behaviour in automotive environments: critical issues in driver interactions with intelligent transport systems. London: Springer; pp. 165-188.

Fuller, R. (2011). *Driver control theory: From task difficulty homeostasis to risk allostasis.* In B. Porter (Ed.), Handbooks of Traffic Psychology. Waltham, MA: Academic Press.

Fuller, R., Bates, H., Gormley, M., Hannigan, B., Stradling, S., Broughton, P., Kinnear, N., & O'Dolan, C. (2008). *The conditions for inappropriate high speed: a review of the research literature from 1995 to 2006.* London: Department of Transport.

Fuller, R., McHugh, C., & Pender, S. (2008). Task difficulty and risk in the determination of driver behaviour. *Revue Européenne De Psychologie Appliquée/European Review of Applied Psychology*, 58(1), 13-21.

Fuller, R., & Santos, J.A. (2002). *Psychology and the highway engineer.* In R. Fuller, & J. A. Santos (Eds.), Human factors for highway engineers. Bingley, UK: Pergamon.

Gabaude, C., Marquié, J., & Obriot-Claudel, F. (2010). Self-regulatory behaviour in the elderly: relationships with aberrant driving behaviours and perceived abilities. *Le Travail Humain,* 73(1), 31-52.

Gabriel, Z., & Bowling, A. (2004). Quality of life from the perspectives of older people. *Ageing and Society,* 24, 675-691.

Gagliardi, C., Marcellini, F., Papa, R., Giuli, C., & Mollenkopf, H. (2010). Associations of personal and mobility resources with subjective well-being among older adults in Italy and Germany. *Archives of Gerontology and Geriatrics,* 50(1), 42-47.

Gibson, J. J., & Crooks, L. E. (1938). A theoretical field-analysis of automobile-driving. *The American Journal of Psychology,* 51(3), 453-471.

Glad, A. (1977). *Requirements regarding drivers: hearing ability*. Oslo: Institute of Transport Economics.

Godthelp, J. (1984). *Studies on human vehicle control.* PhD Thesis, Soesterberg, The Netherlands: Institute for Perception, TNO.

Gopinath B., Schneider, J., McMahon, C. M., Teber, E., Leeder, S. R, Mitchell, P. (2012). Severity of age-related hearing loss is associated with impaired activities of daily living. *Age and Ageing* 41(2):195-200.

Gopinath, B., Schneider, J., Hickson, L., McMahon, C. M., Burlutsky, G., Leeder, S. R., & Mitchell, P. (2012). Hearing handicap, rather than measured hearing impairment, predicts poorer quality of life over 10 years in older adults. *Maturitas,* 72(2), 146-151.

Gordon-Salant, S. (2005). Hearing loss and aging: new research findings and clinical implications. *Rehabilitation Research and Development,* 42(4), 9-23.

Gorman M. (1999) *Development and the rights of older people.* In: Randel, J., German, T., Ewing, D. (Eds.). The ageing and development report: poverty, independence and the world's older people. London: Earthscan Publications; pp 3-21.

Grady, C. (2012). The cognitive neuroscience of ageing. *Nature Reviews Neuroscience,* 13(7), 491-505.

Granick, S., Kleban, M. H. & Weiss, A. D. (1976). Relationships between hearing loss and cognition in normally hearing aged persons. *Journal of Gerontology,* 31(4), 434-440.

Green, K. A., McGwin, G., & Owsley, C. (2013). Associations between visual, hearing, and dual sensory impairments and history of motor vehicle collision involvement of older drivers. *Journal of the American Geriatrics Society,* 61(2), 252-257.

Groeger, J. A. (2000). *Understanding driving: Applying cognitive psychology to a complex everyday task.* London: Routledge.

Grue, E. V., Schroll, M., Jónsson, P. V., Ranhoff, A. H., Noro, A., Finne-Soveri, H., Jonsén, E. (2009). Vision and hearing impairments and their associations with falling and loss of instrumental activities in daily living in acute hospitalized older persons in five Nordic hospitals. *Scandinavian journal of Caring Sciences,* 23(4), 635-643.

Gwyther, H., & Holland, C. (2012). The effect of age, gender and attitudes on self-regulation in driving. *Accident Analysis & Prevention,* 45, 19-28.

Hakamies-Blomqvist, L. (1994). Aging and fatal accidents in male and female drivers. *Social Sciences,* 49(6), 286-290.

Hakamies-Blomqvist, L., & Wahlström, B. (1998). Why do older drivers give up driving? *Accident Analysis & Prevention,* 30(3), 305-312.

Hardin, J., & Hilbe, J. (2003). *Generalized estimating equations.* London: Chapman and Hall/CRC

Hatakka, M., Keskinen, E., Gregersen, N. P., Glad, A., & Hernetkoski, K. (2002). From control of the vehicle to personal self-control; broadening the perspectives to driver education. *Transportation Research Part F: Traffic Psychology and Behaviour,* 5(3), 201-215.

Haustein, S., Sirén, A., Franke E., Pokrieke, E., Alauzet, A., Marin-Lamellet, C., Armoogum, J., O'Neill, D. (2013). *Demographic change and transport.* Final report of WP1:Consol.

Heyl, V., & Wahl, H. W. (2012). Managing daily life with age-related sensory loss: cognitive resources gain in importance. *Psychology and Aging,* 27(2):510-521.

Hitch, G. J., & Halliday, M. S. (1983). Working memory in children. *Philosophical Transactions of the Royal Society of London: Series B,* 302, 325-340.

Hicks, C. B., Tharpe, A. M. (2002). Listening effort and fatigue in school-age children with and without hearing loss. *Journal of Speech, Language, and Hearing Research,* 45, 573-584.

Hicks, T. G. & Wierwille, W. W. (1979). Comparison of five mental workload assessment procedures in a moving-base driving simulator. *Human Factors,* 21(2), 129-143.

Hickson, L., Wood, J., Chaparro, A., Lacherez, P., & Marszalek, R. (2010). Hearing impairment affects older people's ability to drive in the presence of distracters. *Journal of the American Geriatrics Society,* 58(6), 1097-1103.

Hjorthol, R., Levin, L. & Sirén, A. (2010). Mobility in different generations of older persons. The development of daily travel in different cohorts in Denmark, Norway and Sweden. *Journal of Transport Geography,* 18(5), 624-633.

Ho, C., Reed, N., Spence, C. (2006). Assessing the effectiveness of "intuitive" vibrotactile warning signals in preventing front-to-rear-end collisions in a driving simulator. *Accident Analysis and Prevention,* 38, 988-996.

Ho, C., Tan, H. Z., Spence, C. (2005). Using spatial vibrotactile cues to direct visual attention in driving scenes. *Transportation Research Part F: Traffic Psychology and Behaviour,* 8, 397-412.

Holland, C. A. (2009). The relationships between sensory and cognitive decline in older age. *ENT & Audiology News*, 18(4), 94-95.

Holland, C. A., & Rabbitt, P. M. A. (1992). People's Awareness of their age-related sensory and cognitive deficits and the implications for road safety. *Applied Cognitive Psychology,* 6 (3), 217 231.

Hollnagel, E., Nåbo, A., & Lau, I. V. (2003). *A systemic model for driver-in-control.* Paper presented at the Second International Driving Symposium on Human Factors in Driver Assessment, Training and Vehicle Design. Utah, July 21-24.

Howard, C. Q., Maddern, A. J., & Privopoulos, E. P. (2011). Acoustic characteristics for effective ambulance sirens. *Acoustics Australia,* 39, 2-43.

Hua, H. (2014). *Employees with Aided Hearing Impairment: An Interdisciplinary Perspective.* (Doctoral dissertation). Linköping: Linköping University Electronic Press.

Hughes, D., Sapp, G., and Kohler, M. (2006). *Issues in the Intellectual assessment of hearing impaired children.* ERIC Digest. Education Resources Information Center. Available online at: http://www. eric.ed.gov/ERICDocs/data/ericdocs2sql/content_storage_01 /0000019b/80/1b/f1/a4.pdf, pp 1-17. Accessed on September 25, 2014.

Hughes, P. K. & Cole, B. L. (1988). *The effect of attentional demand on eye movement behaviour when driving.* In A. G. Gale, M. H. Freeman, C. M. Haslegrave, P. Smith & S. P. Taylor (Eds.), Vision in vehicles-II (pp. 221–230). Amsterdam: North-Holland.

Hällgren, M., Larsby, B., Lyxell, B., & Arlinger, S. (2001). Evaluation of a cognitive test battery in young and elderly normal-hearing and hearing-impaired persons. *Journal of the American Academy of Audiology,* 12(7), 357-370.

Ivers, R. Q., Mitchell, P., & Cumming, R. G. (1999). Sensory impairment and driving: The Blue Mountains Eye Study. *American Journal of Public Health,* 89(1), 85-87.

Jansen, E., Holte, H., Jung, C., Kahmann, V., Moritz, K., Rietz, C., Rudinger, G., & Weidemann, C. (2001). *Ältere Menschen im künftigen Sicherheitssystem Straße/Fahrzeug/Mensch.* [Senior citizens in the future safety system: street/vehicle/person]. Bremerhaven: Wirtschaftsverlag NW.

Jastak, J. F., & Jastak, S. R. (1964). Short forms of the WAIS and WISC vocabulary subtests. *Journal of Clinical Psychology,* 20(2), 167-199.

Johnston, B. (2008). *Building better surveys: Effective scales.* Best practices. Available at http://www.surveygizmo.com/survey-blog/question-scale-length/. Accessed in August 2014.

Kane, M. J., & Engle, R. W. (2002). The role of prefrontal cortex in working-memory capacity, executive attention, and general fluid intelligence: An individual-differences perspective. *Psychonomic Bulletin & Review* 9(4), 637-671.

Kennedy, Q., Taylor, J. L., Reade, G., & Yesavage, J. A. (2010). Age and expertise effects in aviation decision making and flight control in a flight simulator. *Aviation, Space, and Environmental Medicine,* 81(5), 489.

Kipps, C. M., & Hodges, J. R. (2005). Cognitive assessment for clinicians. *Journal of Neurology Neurosurgery & Psychiatry,* 76 (Suppl 1): 22-30.

Kongsved, S. M., Basnov, M., Holm-Christensen, K., & Hjollund, N. H. (2007). Response rate and completeness of questionnaires: a randomized study of internet versus paper-and-pencil versions. *Journal of Medical Internet Research,* 9(3), e25.

Köpke, S., Deubel, K., Engeln, A., & Schlag, B. (1999). *Mobilitätswahrnehmung und Selbstbild von älteren Autofahrern* [Mobility awareness and self-image of older drivers]. In B. Schlag (Ed.), Empirische Verkehrspsychologie [Empirical traffic psychology]. Lengerich: Pabst Science Publishers; pp. 159-175.

Lehtonen, E., Dahlström, I., Hiltunen, H., & Summala, H. (2012). *On-road visual search and executive functions in elderly drivers.* Paper presented at the International Conference on Traffic and Transport Psychology Groningen, Netherlands August 29-31.

Lewis-Evans, B. (2012). *Testing models of driver behaviour.* (Doctoral dissertation). University of Groningen.

Lewis-Evans, B., de Waard, D., & Brookhuis, K. (2011). Speed maintenance under cognitive load: Implications for theories of driver behaviour. *Accidents Analysis and Prevention,* 43(4), 1497-1507.

Li, K. Z. & Lindenberger, U. (2002). Relations between aging sensory/ sensorimotor and cognitive functions. *Neuroscience and Biobehavioral Reviews,* 26(7), 777-783.

Li, Y., & Perkins, A. (2007). The impact of technological developments on the daily life of the elderly. *Technology in Society,* 29(3), 361-368.

Lidestam, B., Lundqvist, A., & Rönnberg, J. (2010). Concepts from research literature and practical assessment of risk awareness: the Swedish driving test from the perspective of cognitive psychology. *Transportation Research Part F: Traffic Psychology and Behaviour,* 13(6), 409-425.

Liang, K.-Y., & Zeger, S. (1986). Longitudinal data analysis using generalized linear models. *Biometrika* 73(1), 13-22.

Lin, F. R., Ferrucci, L., Metter, E. J., An, Y., Zonderman, A. B., & Resnick, S. M. (2011). Hearing loss and cognition in The Baltimore Longitudinal Study of Aging. *Neuropsychology,* 25 (6), 7637-70.

Lin, F. R., Metter, E. J., O'Brien, R. J., Resnick, S. M., Zonderman, A. B., & Ferrucci, L. (2011). Hearing loss and incident dementia. *Archives of Neurology,* 68(2), 214-220.

Lin, F. R., Yaffe, K., Xia, J., Xue, Q. L., Harris, T. B., Purchase-Helzner, E., Satterfield, S., Ayonayon, H. N., Ferrucci, L., Simonsick, E. M. (2013). Hearing loss and cognitive decline in older adults. *JAMA Internal Medicine,* 173(4), 293-299.

Lin, M. Y., Guttierrez, P. R., Stone, K. L., Yaffe, K., Ensrud, K. E., Fink, H. A. et al.; Study of Osteoporotic Fractures Research Group. (2004). Vision impairment and combined vision and hearing impairment predict cognitive and functional decline in older women. *Journal of the American Geriatrics Society,* 52, 1996-2002.

Lindenberger, U. & Baltes, P. B. (1994). Sensory functioning and intelligence in old age: a strong connection. *Psychology and Aging,* 9, 339-355.

Lindenberger, U., Lövdén, M., Schellenbach, M., Li, S., & Krüger, A. (2008). Psychological Principles of Successful Aging Technologies: A Mini-Review. *Gerontology,* 54, 59-68.

Ljung Aust, M. (2012). *Improving the evaluation process for active safety functions: Addressing key challenges in functional formative evaluation of advanced driver assistance systems.* Thesis, Department of Applied Mechanics, Chalmers University of Technology, Gothenburg, Sweden.

Lundälv J. (2004). Self-reported experiences of incidents and injury events in traffic among hearing impaired people as pedestrians and cyclists. A follow-up study of mobility and use of hearing equipment. *International Journal of Rehabilitation Research,* 27(1):79-80.

Lunner, T. (2003). Cognitive function in relation to hearing aid use. *International Journal of Audiology,* 42 (Suppl 1), S49-S58.

Lyxell, B., Andersson, U., Borg, E., & Ohlsson, I. S. (2003). Working-memory capacity and phonological processing in deafened adults and individuals with a severe hearing impairment. *International Journal of Audiology,* 42, 86-89.

Macintyre, S., Hiscock, R., Kearns, A., & Ellaway, A. (2001). Housing tenure and car access: further exploration of the nature of their relation with health in a UK setting. *Journal of Epidemiology and Community Health,* 52, 657-664.

Magnet, W. (1992). *Empirische Untersuchung zur Kompensationsfrage bei Gehörlosen Autofahrern. Eine Differentielle Analyse der Visuellen Wahrnehmung von Gehörlosen Kraftfahrern* [Empirical examination of compensation made by deaf car drivers. A differential analysis of visual perception by deaf drivers]. Unpublished Dissertation, Universität Innsbruck, Innsbruck.

Marottoli, R., Mendes de Leon, C., Glass, T., Williams, C., Cooney, L. J., Berkman, L. F., & Tinetti, M. (1997). Driving cessation and increased depressive symptoms: prospective evidence from the New Haven EPESE (Established Populations for Epidemiologic Studies of the Elderly). *Journal of the American Geriatrics Society,* 45, 202-206.

Mathers, C., Smith, A., & Concha, M. (2003). *Global burden of hearing loss in the year 2000.* Working paper. Geneva: World Health Organization.

Mayr, U., Spieler, D. H., Kliegl, R. (2001). *Aging and executive control.* New York: Routledge.

McCloskey, L. W., Koepsell, T. D., Wolf, M. E., & Buchner, D. M. (1994). Motor-vehicle collision injuries and sensory impairments of older drivers. *Age and Ageing,* 23(4), 267-273.

McDowd, J. M., & Shaw, R. J. (2000). *Attention and aging: A functional perspective.* In: F. I. M. Craik, & T. A. Salthouse (Eds.), The handbook of aging and cognition, 2nd ed. Mahwah, NJ: Erlbaum; pp. 221-292.

McEvoy, S. P., Stevenson, M. R., & Woodward, M. (2006). The impact of driver distraction on road safety: results from a representative survey in two Australian states. *Injury Prevention,* 12, 242-247.

McHugh, M. L. (2009). The odds ratio: calculation, usage, and interpretation. *Biochemia Medica,* 19(2):120-126.

McKnight, A. J., & Adams, B. B. (1970). *Driver education task analysis. Vol.1: Task descriptions.* Human Resources Research Organization, Alexandria, Virginia. Final Report, Contract No. FH 11-7336.

McRuer, D. T., Allen, R. W., Weir, D. H., & Klein, R. H. (1977). New results in driver steering control models. *Human Factors,* 19, 381-397.

Michon, J. A. (1985). *A critical view of driver behavior models: What do we know, what should we do?* In L. A. Evans, & R. C. Schwing (Eds.), Human behavior and traffic safety. New York: Plenum.

Mitzi M. S., & Johnson, M. (1989). Age differences in decision making: A process methodology for examining strategic information processing. Journal of Gerontology, 45(2), 75-78.

Miyake, A., Friedman, N. P., Emerson, M. J., Witzki, A. H., & Howerter, A. (2000). The unity and diversity of executive functions and their contributions to complex ''frontal lobe'' tasks: A latent variable analysis. *Cognitive Psychology,* 41, 49-100.

Miyake, A. & Shah, P. (1999). *Models of working memory.* Cambridge, UK: Cambridge University Press.

Monsell, S. (1996). *Control of mental processes.* In V. Bruce (Ed.), Unsolved mysteries of the mind: tutorial essays in cognition. Hove, UK: Erlbaum; pp. 93-148.

Monterde-i-Bort, H. (2004). Factorial structure of recklessness: to what extent are older drivers different? *Journal of Safety Research,* 35, 329-335.

Moore, B. C. (1996). Perceptual consequences of cochlear hearing loss and their implications for the design of hearing aids. *Ear and Hearing,* 17(2), 133-161.

Moradi, S., Lidestam, B., Hällgren, M., & Rönnberg, J. (2014). Gated auditory speech perception in elderly hearing aid users and elderly normal-hearing individuals: Effects of hearing impairment and cognitive capacity. *Trends in Hearing*, Jul 31;18. pii: 2331216514545406. doi: 10.1177/ 2331216514545406.

Morris, N., & Jones, D. M. (1990). Memory updating in working memory: the role of the central executive. *British Journal of Psychology,* 81, 111-121.

Mosteller, F. (1968). Association and estimation in contingency tables. *Journal of the American Statistical Association*, 63 (321), 1-28.

Mullen, N., Charlton, J., Devlin., A., & Bédard, M. (2001). *Simulator validity: Behaviors observed on the simulator and on the road.* In D. L. Fisher, M. Rizzo, J. K. Caird, & J. D. Lee (Eds.), Driving simulation for engineering, medicine and psychology. Florida: Taylor and Francis.

Nakeva von Mentzer, C. (2014). *Rethinking Sound: Computer-assisted reading intervention with a phonics approach for deaf and hard of hearing children using cochlear implants or hearing aids.* (Doctoral dissertation). Linköping: Linköping University Electronic Press.

Näätänen, R., & Summala, H. (1974). A model for the role of motivational factors in drivers' decision-making. *Accident Analysis & Prevention,* 6(3-4), 243-261.

Neisser, U. (1976). *Cognition and reality: Principles and implications of cognitive psychology:* New York: W.H. Freeman.

Nilsson, L. (1993). *Contributions and limitations of simulator studies to driver behaviour research.* In A. A. M. Parkes, & S. Franzen (Eds.), Driving future vehicles: Taylor & Francis; pp. 401-407.

O'Brien, S. (2009) *Eye tracking in translation process research: Methodological challenges and solutions.* In: I. M. Mees, F. Alves, & S. Gopferich (Eds.), Methodology, technology and innovation in translation process research: A tribute to Arnt Lykke Jakobsen. Copenhagen Studies in Language, vol. 38. Copenhagen: Samfundslitteratur; pp. 251-266.

O'Donnell, R. D. & Eggemeier, F. T. (1986). *Workload assessment methodology.* In K. R. Boff, L. Kaufman, & J. P. Thomas (Eds.), Handbook of perception and human performance, vol. II, Cognitive processes and performance. New York: Wiley; pp. 42/1-42/49.

O'Hanlon, J. F. (1984). Driving performance under the influence of drugs: rationale for, and application of, a new test. *British Journal of Clinical Pharmacology*, 18, 121S-129S.

O'Hanlon, J. F., Haak, T. W., Blaauw, G. J. & Riemersma, J. B. J. (1982). Diazepam impairs lateral position control in highway driving. *Science,* 217, 79-80.

Ohta, H., & Komatsu, H. (1991). *Speed perception in driving*. Vision in vehicles, vol. III. Amsterdam: Elsevier Science Publishers; pp. 415-426.

Owsley, C., Ball, K., McGwin, G., Sloane, M. E., Roenker, D. L., White, M. F. et al. (1998). Visual processing impairment and risk of motor vehicle crash among older adults. *Journal of the American Medical Association,* 279(14), 1083-1088.

Parasuraman, R., & Riley, V. (1997) Humans and automation: use, misuse, disuse, abuse. *Human Factors,* 39(2), 230-253.

Pearson, J. D., Morrell, C. H., Gordon-Salant, S., Brant, L. J., Metter, E. J., Klein, L. L., & Fozard, J. L. (1995). Gender differences in a longitudinal-study of age-associated hearing-loss. *Journal of the Acoustical Society of America,* 97(2), 1196-1205.

Pelli, D. G., Robson, J. G., & Wilkins, A. J. (1988). The design of a new letter chart for measuring contrast sensitivity. *Clinical Vision Sciences,* 2, 187-199.

Peters, B., & Nielsen, B. (2007). A strategy aiming to compensate degraded abilities among elderly drivers. *11th International Conference on Mobility and Transport for Elderly and Disabled Persons,* Montreal, Canada.

Peters, B., & Nilsson, L. (2006). *Modelling the driver in control.* In P. Cacciabue (Ed.), Modelling driver behaviour in automotive environments: Critical issues in driver interactions with intelligent transport systems. London: Springer.

Peters C. A., Potter J. F., & Scholer S. G. (1988). Hearing impairment as a predictor of cognitive decline in dementia. *Journal of the American Geriatriatrics Society,* 36(11):981-986.

Phillips, N. A., & Lesperance, D. (2003). Breaking the waves: age differences in electrical brain activity when reading text with distractors. *Psychology and Aging,* 18(1), 126-139.

Picard, M., Girard, S.A., Courteau, M., Leroux, T., Larocque, R., Turcotte, F., et al. (2008). Could driving safety be compromised by noise exposure at work and noise-induced hearing loss? *Traffic Injury Prevention,* 9(5), 489-499.

Pichora-Fuller, M. K., & Singh, G. (2006). Effects of age on auditory and cognitive processing: implications for hearing aid fitting and audiologic rehabilitation. *Trends in Amplification,* 10(1), 29-59.

Rajalin, S., Hassel, S. O., & Summala, H. (1997). Close-following drivers on two-lane highways. *Accident Analysis & Prevention,* 29(6), 723-729.

Ranney, T. (1994) Models of driving behavior: a review of their evolution. *Accident Analysis & Prevention,* 26(6), 733-750.

Pohlmann, S. & Traenkle, U. (1994). Orientation in road traffic. Age-related differences using an in-vehicle navigation system and a conventional map. *Accident Analysis & Prevention,* 26, 689-702.

Reitan, R. (1986). *Trail making test.* Manual for administration and scoring. Tuscon, AZ: Neuropsychological Laboratory.

Repovs, G. & Baddeley, A. (2006). The multi-component model of working memory: explorations in experimental cognitive psychology. *Neuroscience Special Issue,* 139, 5-21.

Riediger, M., Li, S. C., & Lindenberger, U. (2006). Selection, optimization, and compensation as developmental mechanisms of adaptive resource allocation: Review and preview. *Handbook of the psychology of aging,* 6, 289-313.

Rimmer, J. (2006). Use of the ICF in identifying factors that impact participation in physical abilities/rehabilitation among people with disabilities. *Disability and Rehabilitation,* 28, 1087-1095.

Rimmö, P.-A., & Hakamies-Blomqvist, L. (2002). Older drivers' aberrant driving behaviour, impaired activity, and health as reasons for self-imposed driving limitations. *Transportation Research Part F: Traffic Psychology and Behaviour,* 5, 345-360.

Risacher, S. L., Wudunn, D., Pepin, S. M., MaGee, T. R., McDonald, B. C., Flashman, L. A. et al. (2013). Visual contrast sensitivity in Alzheimer's disease, mild cognitive impairment, and older adults with cognitive complaints. *Neurobiology of Aging,* 34(4):1133-1144.

Roebuck, J. (1979). When does old age begin? The evolution of the English definition. *Journal of Social History*, 12(3):416-428.

Roth, T. N., Hanebuth, D., & Probst, R. (2001). Prevalence of age-related hearing loss in Europe: a review. *European Archives of Oto-Rhino-Laryngology,* 268(8), 1101-1107.

Rothe, J. P. (1990). *The safety of elderly drivers*. London: Transaction Publishers.

Rouse, W. B., Edwards, S. L. & Hammer, J. M. (1993). Modelling the dynamics of mental workload and human performance in complex systems. *IEEE transactions on systems, man, and cybernetics,* 23, 1662-1671.

Rumar, K. (1988). Collective risk but individual safety. *Ergonomics,* 31(4), 507-518.

Rönnberg, J. (1990). Cognitive and communicative function: the effects of chronological age and "handicap age". *European Journal of Cognitive Psychology,* 2, 253-273.

Rönnberg, J., Danielsson, H., Rudner, M., Arlinger, S., Sternang, O., Wahlin, A., & Nilsson, L. G. (2011). Hearing loss is negatively related to episodic and semantic long-term memory but not to short-term memory. *Journal of Speech Language and Hearing Research,* 54(2), 705-726.

Rönnlund, M., Nyberg, L., Bäckman, L., & Nilsson, L. G. (2005). Stability, growth, and decline in adult life span development of declarative memory: cross-sectional and longitudinal data from a population based study. *Psychology and Aging,* 20(1), 3-18.

Salthouse, T. A., Babcock, R. L. (1991). Decomposing adult age-differences in working memory. *Developmental Psychology,* 27(5), 763-776.

Salthouse, T. A. (1996). The processing-speed theory of adult age differences in cognition. *Psychological Review.* 103: 403-428.

Salvucci D. D. (2006) Modeling Driver Behavior in a Cognitive Architecture. *Human Factors,* 48 (2), 362-380

Sandberg, U. (2003). *The multi-coincidence peak around 1000 Hz in tyre/road noise spectra. Paper presented at the Euronoise.* May, 19-21, Naples.

Saremi, A., & Stenfelt, S. (2013). Effect of metabolic presbyacusis on cochlear responses: a simulation approach using a physiologically-based model. *Journal of the Acoustic Society of America,* 134(4), 2833-2851.

Schmolz, W. (1987). Die Bedeutung des Hoehrens im Verkehr. [The effect of hearing in traffic]. *Polizei Verkehr Technik,* 32(11), 379-380.

Schneider, B. A., Pichora-Fuller, M. K., & Daneman, M. (2010). *Effects of senescent changes in audition and cognition on spoken language comprehension.* In S. Gordon-Salant, R. R. Frisina, R. R. Fay, & A. Popper(Eds.), The aging auditory system. New York: Springer.

Schneider, J., Gopinath, B., Karpa, M. J., McMahon, C. M., Rochtchina, E., Leeder, S. R., & Mitchell, P. (2010). Hearing loss impacts on the use of community and informal supports. *Age and Ageing,* 39(4), 458-464.

Selander, H., Lee, H. C., Johansson, K., & Falkmer, T. (2011). Older drivers: on-road and off-road test results. *Accidents Analysis and Prevention,* 43 (4). 1348-1354.

Shinar, D. (2007). *Traffic safety and human behavior.* Oxford: Elsevier.

Sirén, A., & Hakamies-Blomqvist, L. (2004). Private car as the grand equaliser? Demographic factors and mobility in Finnish men and women aged 65+. *Transportation Research Part F: Traffic Psychology and Behaviour,* 7(2), 107-118.

Sirén, A. & Hakamies-Blomqvist, L. (2009). Mobility and well-being in old age. *Topics in Geriatric Rehabilitation,* 25(1), 3-11.

Sternberg, S. (1966). High-speed scanning in human memory. *Science,* 153, 652-654.

Stevens, G., Flaxman, S., Brunskill, E., Mascarenhas, M., Mathers, C. D., & Finucane, M. (2013). Global and regional hearing impairment prevalence: an analysis of 42 studies in 29 countries. *European Journal of Public Health,* 23(1), 146-152.

Sullivan, K. A., Smith, S. S., Horswill, M. S., & Lurie-Beck, J. K. (2011). Older adults' safety perceptions of driving situations: towards a new driving self-regulation scale. *Accident Analysis & Prevention,* 43(3), 1003-1009.

Summala, H. (2005). *Traffic psychology theories: Towards understanding driving behaviour and safety efforts.* In G. Underwood (Ed.), Traffic and Transport Psychology. Amsterdam: Elsevier; pp. 383-394,

Summala, H. (2007). *Towards understanding motivational and emotional factors in driver behaviour: Comfort through satisficing.* In C. Cacciabue (Ed.), Modelling Driver Behaviour in Automotive Environments. London: Springer; pp. 189-207.

Summala, H., Etholén, T., Leino, N., Niskakangas, M., Laine, M. & Saarinen, S. (2008). *FR-TMT: Visuospatial (working) memory in a computerized Trail-Making test.* Poster presented at the Psykologia 2008 Congress, August 20-22, Helsinki.

Teng E. L., Chui H. C. (1987) The Modified Mini-Mental State (3MS) Examination. *Journal of Clinical Psychiatry,* 48(8):314-318.

Thomas, P. D., Hunt, W. C., Garry, P. J., Hood, R. B., Goodwin, J. M. & Goodwin, J. S. (1983). Hearing acuity in a healthy elderly population: effects on emotional, cognitive, and social status. *Journal of Gerontology,* 38, 321-325.

Tun, P. A., McCoy, S., & Wingfield, A. (2009) Aging, hearing acuity, and the attentional costs of effortful listening. *Psychology and Aging,* 24(3), 761-766.

Vaa, T. (2003). *Survival or deviance? A model for driver behaviour.* (TOI report 666/2003). Oslo: Institute of Transport Economics.

Vaa, T. (2007). *Modelling driver behaviour on basis of emotions and feelings: Intelligent transport systems and behavioural adaptations.* In C. Cacciabue (Ed.), Modelling driver behaviour in automotive environments. London: Springer; pp. 208-232.

Vaa, T. (2011). *Proposing a driver behaviour model based on emotions and feelings: Exploring the boundaries of perception and learning.* In M. Regan, T. Victor & J. Lee (Eds.), Driver distraction and inattention: advances in research and countermeasures. Farnham, UK: Ashgate Publishing.

Vaa, T., Glad, A., & Sagberg, F. (2000). *Developing a model of driver behaviour: Introductory working papers.* (TOI report 503/2000). Oslo: Institute of Transport Economics.

Valentijn S. A., van Boxtel M. P., van Hooren S. A., Bosma H., Beckers H. J., Ponds R. W., & Jolles J. (2005). Change in sensory functioning predicts change in cognitive functioning: results from a 6-year follow-up in the Maastricht Aging Study. *Journal of the American Geriatrics Society* 53(3), 374-380.

Van der Linden, M., Brédart, S., & Beerten, A. (1994). Age-related differences in updating working memory. *British Journal of Psychology,* 85, 145-152.

Van der Linden, M., Hupet, M., Feyereisen, P., Schelstraete, M., Bestgen, M., Bruyer, G. L., Abdessadek, E. A., & Seron., X. (1999). Cognitive mediators of age-related differences in language comprehension and verbal processing. *Aging, Neuropsychology, and Cognition,* 6, 32-55.

Van Erp, J. B. F., & van Veen, H. A. H. C. (2004). Vibrotactile in-vehicle navigation system. *Transportation Research Part F: Traffic Psychology and Behaviour*, 7, 247-256.

Verhaeghen, P., Cerella, J., Bopp, K. L., & Basak, C. (2005). *Aging and varieties of cognitive control: a review of meta-analyses on resistance to interference, coordination, and task switching, and experimental exploration of age-sensitivity in the newly identified process of focus switching.* In: R. W. Engle, G. Sedek, U. von Hecker, & D. N. McIntosh (Eds), Cognitive limitations in aging and psychopathology. New York: Cambridge University Press; pp. 160-189.

Verhaeghen, P., Steitz, D. W., Sliwinski, M. J., & Cerella, J. (2003). Aging and dual-task performance: a meta-analysis. *Psychology and Aging,* 18, 443-460.

Vreeken, H. L., van Rens, G., Knol, D. L., van Reijen, N. A., Kramer, S. E., Festen, M. J., & van Nispen, R. M. A. (2013). Dual sensory loss: a major age-related increase of comorbid hearing loss and hearing aid ownership in visually impaired adults. *Geriatrics and Gerontology International.* Available at http://www.biomedcentral.com/1471-2318/13/84. Accessed on September 25, 2014.

Wallhagen, M. I. (2010). The stigma of hearing loss. *Gerontologist,* 50(1), 66-75.

Wechsler D. (1981). *Manual for the Wechsler Adult Intelligence Scale-revised.* New York: Psychological Corp.

Wickens, C. D., & Hollands, J. G. (1999). *Engineering Psychology and Human Performance* (3nd ed.). New York: Harper Collins.

Wilson, G. F. & Eggemeier, F. T. (1991). *Psychophysiological assessment of workload in multi-task environments.* In D. L. Damos (Ed.), Multiple-task performance. London: Taylor & Francis; pp. 329–360.

World Health Organization (WHO). (2001). *International Classification of Functioning, Disability and Health (ICF).* Geneva: World Health Organization.

Wu, Y. H., Aksan, N., Rizzo, M., Stangl, E., Zhang, X., & Bentler, R. (2014). Measuring listening effort: driving simulator versus simple dual-task paradigm. *Ear and Hearing,* doi: 10.1097/AUD.0000000000000079.

Wu, Y. H., Stangl, E., Bentler, R., & Stanziola, R. W. (2013). The effect of hearing aid technologies on listening in an automobile. *Journal of Clinical Experimental Neuropsychology of the American Academy of Audiology,* 24(6), 474-485.

In: Handbook of Hearing Disorders Research
Editor: Charlotte Hailee Atkinson
ISBN: 978-1-63463-654-4

Chapter 2

Occupational Exposure to Ototoxic Chemicals

M. P. Gatto[1], R. C. Bonanni[1], G. Tranfo[1], E. Strafella[2], L. Santarelli[2] and M. Gherardi[1]

[1]INAIL, Department of Occupational and Environmental Medicine, Epidemiology and Hygiene, Monte Porzio Catone (RM), Italy

[2]Marche Polytechnic University, PhD School, Safety and Health at the Workplace, Ancona, Italy

Abstract

There is a growing awareness that a variety of different chemical substances can cause hearing damage in humans. The literature of the last decade on the effect of different chemical compounds on the human auditory system has been reviewed with reference to the exposure in the workplace. Scientific evidence has emerged that the exposure to styrene, p-xylene, solvent mixtures and lead may be a cause of hearing loss. For these substances the number of studies is relatively large and a variety of approaches have been undertaken to test their effect on the auditory system. For other chemical substances, for example certain metals such as mercury, cadmium and arsenic, and some neurotoxic pesticides, the available data indicate a possible ototoxic action, although in some cases only when in combination with noise. A number of critical aspects have been noticed: firstly, this review highlights the need to consider the possible synergistic effect of the interactions between different ototoxic agents, primarily the co-exposure to noise. These interactions are complex and difficult to predict, since synergistic, additive and sub-additive effects have to be contemplated. Then, the individual variability of exposed subjects, due to genetic differences, personal clinical histories, and occupational/ environmental exposures cannot be disregarded. Finally, there are conceptual differences among the studies in the definition of hearing loss, which may partly account for the different prevalence values found in the examined documents. In conclusion, it is suggested to adopt the precautionary principle, while awaiting, on one hand, a stronger evidence on the ototoxicity of some classes of chemicals, particularly for exposures at low doses, and, on the other hand, new scientific studies on the effects of the interaction between physical and chemical agents on the hearing loss that are a priority in future research needs.

Introduction

The problem of hearing loss, with the consequences resulting from this disease, is of great concern in the medical community. Deafness is one of the most widespread, costly and poorly understood disabilities in the world. According to the World Health Organization (WHO) about 250 million people have disabling hearing loss and two-thirds of them live in the developing world. Millions of people progressively lose their most important means of communication and became socially isolated, especially in the later years of their life (Gatto et al., 2013). Previous studies have shown that hearing deficits can also contribute to occupational injury, although most of these studies evaluated traumatic injury (Hétu et al., 1995; Sprince et al., 2003; Choi et al., 2005). Even if age-related changes, noise exposure and head trauma are the most common causes of damage to cochlear hair cells, several other factors may also cause hearing loss. Since the early 1980s, indeed, some chemical agents have been investigated in order of their potential ototoxic properties in humans. An ototoxic substance is any chemical or mixture that may impair the structures and/or the function of the inner ear (auditory plus vestibular apparatus) and the connected neural pathways; those substances that instead impair hearing and balance by affecting mainly the central or peripheral nervous system are considered neurotoxic. Ototoxic agents are generally divided into two groups, occupational and non-occupational chemicals: this study focused on the first one, even if a brief mention about other xenobiotics that may affect the auditory system is essential. Drugs are considered the main non-occupational substances that may damage hearing: these include, for example, antibiotics, with a place of absolute importance for the aminoglycosides, diuretics, and salicylates, certain antineoplastics such as cisplatin and carboplatin, and anti-malarial medications. In addition, despite the presence of a considerable uncertainty, some lifestyle habits, such as cigarette smoking and alcohol consumption, are also believed to be ototoxic. The classes of compounds discussed in this chapter include organic solvents, metals, pesticides, and other chemicals, including polychlorinated biphenyls and asphyxiants, grouped in a separate class.

Organic Solvents

There is ample scientific evidence that the exposure to several solvents, either alone or in concert with noise exposure, has ototoxic effects. The aromatic solvents of the alkylbenzene family are the largest group among the solvents that have been found to affect the auditory system. Animal models have demonstrated that the relative ototoxicity may vary among the aromatic solvents (Gagnaire & Langlais, 2005). A tentative ranking of increasing ototoxocity for aromatic solvents could be proposed on the basis of cochlea morphological investigation and histological hair cell losses as: α-methylstyrene, trans-β-methylstyrene = toluene ≤ p-xylene < n-propylbenzene < styrene = ethylbenzene < allylbenzene. No relationship between the degree of ototoxicity and the lipophilic properties of the ototoxic agents as expressed by the octanol/water partition coefficients was observed. However, correlations between some structural properties and ototoxicity were observed. A single side-chain on the aromatic ring, except with p-xylene, is essential for ototoxicity. The other aromatic solvents with two side-chains were not ototoxic. When the saturated side-chain was branched (isopropylbenzene, isobutylbenzene, sec-butylbenzene, tert-butylbenzene), no ototoxicity was found. Also the saturation and the number of carbon atoms in the side-chain are of importance. The ototoxic potency increases when the length of the saturated side-chain extended from one carbon atom to two carbon atoms. Of the xylene isomers, p-xylene showed ototoxic effects whereas o-xylene and m-xylene did not (Maguin et al., 2006). Moreover, branching of the unsaturated chain (α-methylstyrene and trans-β-methylstyrene) decreased the ototoxicity of styrene. Finally, some aliphatic solvents, such as n-hexane and n-heptane, as well as trichloroethylene and carbon disulphide, have effects on neurons in the central nervous system, and consequently are supposed to also affect the auditory system (Morata, 1989; Nylén et al., 1994; Simonsen & Lund, 1995; Vyskocil et al., 2008a.b).

Styrene

Styrene is used in the production of plastics, rubber, and resins. Several occupational studies have been investigated the effects of styrene on the auditory system alone or in concert with noise. Reviewed papers were cross-sectional epidemiological studies or occupational health cohort studies. Exposure assessment was based on styrene measurements in the breathing zone, usually also supported by the biological monitoring of its urinary metabolites. In many studies, lifetime exposure to both styrene and noise was calculated using company records and questionnaire data. The results are equivocal. Some studies (Johnson et al., 2006; Mascagni et al., 2007; Morata et al., 2011; Sisto et al., 2013) claimed to have demonstrated styrene-induced hearing loss in industrial populations, also with synergism between styrene and noise, but others (Hoffmann et al., 2006; Triebig et al., 2009) have indicated no ototoxic effects of styrene exposure. Johnson et al. (2006) studied the health effects in 313 workers exposed to noise (> 85dBA) and styrene and to styrene alone (noise < 85 dBA). Workers exposed to styrene alone or in combination with noise resulted to have significantly poorer pure-tone thresholds in the high-frequency range (3-8 kHz) than the control, noise-only exposed workers and non occupationally noise-exposed. In a smaller study, hearing thresholds of 32 workers in a fiberglass reinforced industry were compared to 60 unexposed control subjects (Mascagni et al., 2007). Twenty-four of the exposed subjects had slightly but significantly higher thresholds at all frequencies (except at 8 kHz on the right ear). The study confirmed the results from earlier studies with larger population that styrene alone can cause a slightly elevated hearing threshold (Muijser et al., 1988; Morioka et al., 1999; Sliwińska-Kowalska et al., 2003). Similar findings were reported by a large cross-sectional study on styrene-exposed workers from Sweden, Finland, and Poland (Morata et al., 2011). Among the important results obtained from this multicenter study, such as the corroboration of association between styrene exposure and hypoacusis, the authors observed that noise exposure from 80 to 84 dBA did not have a significant effect on hearing, except when in combination with styrene. In a recent study Sisto et al. (2013) evaluated the ototoxic effect of styrene by means of otoacoustic emissions, used as biomarkers of mild cochlear damage. The authors found a significant correlation between the otoacoustic emission levels and the concentration of the styrene urinary metabolites. Besides, on a subsample of styrene exposed subjects with low exposure to noise and short exposure lifetime, cochlear functionality degradation has been evidenced, manifesting itself with a significant reduction of the otoacoustic signals. In contrast, other studies failed to find any effect of styrene on hearing thresholds. An investigation on 32 workers of a boat building factory found no consistent association and only few isolated correlations between the parameters of hearing acuity and exposure indices (Hoffmann et al., 2006). No clear ototoxic effects were also reported by Triebig et al. (2009). The study examined associations between occupational styrene exposure and impairment of hearing function of a group of workers from a boat building plant. With the exception at frequencies of 1,000 and 1,500 Hz, no dose-response relationship between threshold and exposure data was found. In conclusion, there is some suggestion of a likely ototoxic effect of styrene exposure, but hearing dysfunction deficits, in particular at low concentrations, have not been demonstrated by scientifically reliable argument. Further studies in humans are necessary to clarify this question.

Toluene

Toluene has a number of industrial uses as solvent, carrier, or thinner in the paint, rubber, printing, cosmetic, adhesives and resin industries, as a starting material for the synthesis of other chemicals and as a constituent of fuels. Information gained from animal studies support the observations in humans that toluene can be ototoxic (Pryor & Howd, 1986; Johnson et al., 1988; Sullivan et al., 1989; Li et al., 1992) and demonstrate that toluene exposure can aggravate auditory degeneration in genetically predisposed mice. The data on the ototoxic effect of toluene in humans originate mainly from case reports of acute toluene poisoning. In studies focused on the voluntary inhalation of toluene, severe hearing loss in the central auditory pathways was reported (Ryback, 1992; Morata et al., 1994). Two studies on association between auditory damage and occupational exposure to toluene were identified in the literature of the last 10 years. Chang et al. (2006) described hearing impairment from simultaneous exposure to toluene and noise in 174 workers at an adhesive materials manufacturing plant. Diametrically opposite conclusions have been reached by Schaper et al. (2008). In a five year follow-up study, 333 rotogravure printers exposed to a relatively high level of toluene in the printing area were compared with those exposed to a low level of toluene in the end-processing area. No toluene exposure-related variables (duration, level, urine metabolites) were found to be significant in the logistic regression model. To sum up, toluene may be associated with hearing impairment when the exposure reaches a certain level (Chang et al., 2006); the risk effect may not be observed when the level is lower than 50 ppm (Schaper et al., 2008). However, more studies are needed to confirm these findings.

Xylenes

Xylenes are found in various solvent mixtures, including paints, varnishes, and thinners; they are also used in histology laboratories. Several studies have been compared the ototoxicity of three xylene isomers (Pryor et al., 1987; Cappaert et al., 1999, 2000; Campo et al., 2001; Gagnaire et al., 2001; Maguin et al., 2006). Unlike o-xylene and m-xylene, an ototoxic effect was observed after a sub chronic p-xylene exposure.

In 2008, Draper & Bamiou presented a case-study of a patient with auditory neuropathy after exposure to xylene, and in the absence of any other risk factor. More recently, in a study on a group of 30 medical laboratory workers, Fuente et al. (2013) found significant different ABR latencies for xylene-exposed workers than non-exposed workers.

Dichloromethane

Dichloromethane is a widely used organic solvent in a diverse range of industries such as metals and plastics, electronics, pesticides and textiles. The effects of dichloromethane on the auditory system have been debated in a recent study conducted by Bonfiglioli et al. (2014). The authors reported the case of a transient bilateral hypoacusis after acute exposure to dichloromethane, suggesting a possible ototoxic effect of this solvent.

Trichloroethylene

Trichloroethylene is primarily used as a grease remover, but is also used as a dry-cleaning agent and as a chemical intermediary in the production of paints, waxes, pesticides, and other products, such as adhesive and lubricants.

In animal models, exposure to high concentrations of trichloroethylene has been shown to disrupt cochlear sensory hair and spiral ganglion cells, mainly in the middle turn, as well, i.e. the auditory nervous pathways within the cochlea (Prasher et al., 2004; Albee et al., 2006). In a review of the literature on the effects of low-level exposure to trichloroethylene on the auditory system, Vyskocil et al. (2008b) found no convincing scientific evidence of trichloroethylene induced hearing losses in workers. No human study on the interaction between occupational trichloroethylene exposure and noise was found.

Carbon Disulphide

Despite the usage of carbon disulfide (CS_2) is strictly controlled by legislation, because of its physico-chemical and toxicological properties, it is still widely used in various sectors such as in the textile industry for the production of rayon fibers and in industrial applications, mainly in tires and other reinforced rubber articles. Carbon disulphide is known to be a neurotoxicant and in some previous studies the effects on the auditory system in workers have been interpreted as a consequence of the known central nervous system (CNS) toxicity of the substance.

Gelbke et al. (2009), in a review of literature on CS_2 health effects, suggest that hearing deficits will only occur at relatively high carbon disulfide exposures, and there may be an interaction between CS_2 exposure and ambient noise levels. The authors concluded that the studies with highest utility support that an Occupational Exposure Limits (OEL) of 10 ppm "may be low enough to protect workers from significant aggravated hearing impairment due to CS_2 exposure in a noisy working condition" (Chang et al., 2003). However, the number of investigations on electroencephalogram (EEG) alterations and especially on the audio-vestibular system is too small to come to a final decision. Audiometric studies in workers under defined long-term exposure conditions would be helpful in this respect.

Solvent Mixtures

Several other organic solvents, such as ethylbenzene, n-hexane, methyl ethyl ketone (MEK), ethyl acetate, butyl acetate, have been hypothesized to impair hearing. These chemicals are rarely present separately in workplaces, but mostly as solvent mixtures. Over the recent literature, five occupational studies examining the relationship between solvent mixtures and hearing impairment have been identified. A variety of workplaces was investigated, including paint and lacquer industry, petroleum refineries, aviation industry, shipyards, and work environments exposed to jet fuel. Kim et al., (2005) studied hearing impairments as consequence of simultaneous exposure to noise and mixed solvents in the aviation industry. The major components in the solvent mixtures were methyl ethyl ketone, toluene, xylene, and methyl isobutyl ketone. The study found a prevalence of hearing loss of 54.9% among workers exposed to noise and mixed solvents simultaneously; 17.1% among workers exposed only to noise; 27.8% among workers only exposed to a solvent mixture; and 6% among non-exposed workers. Relative risks were estimated to be 4.3 for the noise-only group, 8.1 for the noise and solvents group, and 2.6 for the solvents mixture group. In a similar study conducted by Kaufman et al. (2005), the exposure to jet fuels, containing several solvents such as n-hexane, n-heptanes, toluene, and xylenes, was found to increase the odds ratio when it is combined with noise exposure during the first twelve years of exposure. The effects of jet fuel exposure on hearing were found statistically non-significant for more than 12 years of combined noise and jet fuel exposure, suggesting a plateau effect for jet fuel exposure and/or that the noise-induced hearing loss may become more important for those continuing to have exposure to both agents. In the last decade two studies on the association between hearing impairment and the exposure to solvent mixtures and noise were published by Sliwinska-Kowalska et al. In the first study (Sliwinska-Kowalska et al., 2004), the authors compared the hearing impairments of 701 dockyard workers (517 noise and organic solvent mixture exposed and 184 noise only exposed) with 205 control subjects not exposed to either noise or solvents. The odds ratio of hearing loss resulted significantly increased by about three times in the noise-only group and by almost five times in the noise and solvent group. In the second study (Sliwinska-Kowalska et al., 2005) hearing disabilities of 1117 workers exposed to both mixtures of solvents (xylene, styrene, n-hexane and toluene) and noise were confronted with 66 workers exposed to noise only and 157 controls. A positive linear relationship was found between exposure to solvents and hearing thresholds at high frequencies. All solvent exposures were found to be associated with hearing impairment, with the lowest odds ratios in the solvent-mixture-exposed group (xylene as the main component), and the highest in the n-hexane and toluene exposed group. The authors also indicated that additional deterioration of hearing at 8 kHz could be caused by co-exposure to solvents and noise. More recently, Fuente et al. (2011) conducted an investigation on central auditory functioning in normal hearing, solvent-exposed subjects (n=46) compared to normal-hearing, non-exposed subjects (n=46). Although all subjects had normal-hearing thresholds, solvent-exposed participants exhibited significantly poorer hearing thresholds in comparison to non-exposed subjects. Data were in agreement with results from a study conducted in 2007, in which Fuente et al. demonstrated that solvents were significantly associated with poorer pure-tone thresholds, lower amplitudes of transient evoked otoacoustic emissions (TEOAEs), and poorer results for central auditory functioning tests.

In summary, the literature data revealed the increased risk of hearing loss in workers exposed to organic solvent mixture only, and well documented the potentiating of harmful effects of combined exposure to solvents and noise. Hearing impairment is mainly observed in high frequencies, but lower frequencies can also be involved. Some studies have revealed that pure-tone audiometry might be insufficient to differentiate between noise and chemical ototoxic effects (Sliwinska-Kowalska et al., 2004; Fuente et al., 2008, 2011). Finally, it must be emphasized that current exposure limits for solvents, established separately for each single chemical, are probably not effective in hearing protection when they are mixed.

Table 1. Occupational studies on auditory effects of solvents exposure

Substance [CAS]	Structure	ACGIH TLV-TWA (STEL)*	Industrial Uses	Weight of evidence	References
Styrene [100-42-5]	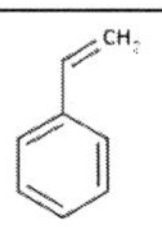	20 (40)	*Fiberglass*, rubber, plastic, insulation.	O/PO	Johnson et al., 2006; Hoffmann et al., 2006; Mascagni et al., 2007; Triebig et al., 2009; Morata et al., 2011; Sisto et al., 2013
Toluene [108-88-3]	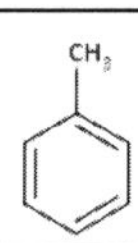	20	Solvent of paints, lacquers, thinners, glues and industrial feedstock	O/PO	Chang et al., 2006; Schaper et al., 2008
p-xylene [106-42-3]	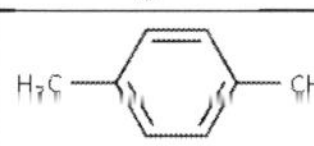	100 (150)	Solvent in leather, rubber and printing industries	O/PO	Draper & Bamiou, 2008; Fuente et al., 2010
Dichloromethane [75-09-2]	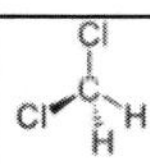	50	In paint removers, in manufacturing process of film coatings, as aerosol spray propellant.	NC	Bonfiglioli et al., 2014
Trichloroethylene [79-01-6]	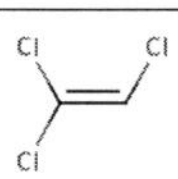	10 (25)	Degreaser in metal industry and in chemical laundries.	NE	Vyskocil et al., 2008
Carbon Disulphide [75-15-0]	S=C=S	1 (3.1)	Man-made cellulosic fibers, tires and other reinforced rubber articles.	PO	Gelbke et al., 2009
Solvent mixtures	Ethylbenzene, n-hexane, carbon disulfide, methyl ethyl ketone (MEK), ethyl acetate, butyl acetate		In dry cleaning, as paint thinners, and glue solvents	O/PO	Sliwinska-Kowalska et al., 2004, 2005; Kaufman et al., 2005; Kim et al., 2005; Fuente et al., 2008, 2011

CAS: Chemical Abstracts Service; TLV: Threshold Limit Value – TWA: time-weighted average; STEL: Short-Term Exposure Limit; O: ototoxic substance, PO: possibly ototoxic substance, NC: nonconclusive, NE: no evidence. *Values in Parts Per Million (ppm).

Metals

In animal studies, metals such as lead, mercury, cadmium, and manganese are reported to impair inner ear cells, leading to auditory function disorders (Yamamura et al., 1989; Lasky et al., 1995; Ozcaglar et al., 2001; Jones et al., 2008; Kim et al., 2008). Human studies are sparse, but there are some data supporting their effect on auditory system (Chuang et al., 2007; Shargorodsky et al., 2011; Choi et al., 2012; Saunders et al., 2013). The interaction with the noise has been poorly studied either in animals or in humans. Some of the ototoxic metals are discussed in the following section.

Lead

Lead can be found in various workplaces, such as constructions, wholesale trade, industries involved in the manufacture of ammunition, batteries, chemical compounds, explosives, glassware, and metal products. OSHA estimates that approximately 804,000 workers in general industry and an additional 838,000 workers in construction are potentially exposed to lead. Experimental studies on animal models suggest that lead exposure induces degeneration in the inner ear receptor cells and latency in auditory nerve conduction velocity (Yamamura et al., 1989; Lasky et al., 1995). There are contradictory findings on hearing loss from human lead exposure. Several epidemiological studies on lead-exposed workers whose blood lead levels have been related to audiological findings, suggest a probable ototoxic effect for this metal (Chuang et al., 2007; Hwang et al., 2009; Galal et al., 2011). The study conducted by Galal et al. (2011) on a sample of 61 lead-exposed and 50 non-exposed found a significant correlation r=0.7 between blood lead levels and binaural hearing impairment. Similar results were observed on 412 workers exposed to low-level lead in a steel plant (Hwang, 2009). In addition of results on lead ototoxicity, Chuang et al., (2007) found that selenium was inversely associated with hearing thresholds, and it may be considered an antagonist to Pb ototoxicity. On the contrary, Counter et al., (2009) were unable to substantiate this in their study on a group of subjects with a history of chronic exposure from occupational Pb glazing. In the past it has also been suggested that lead exposure results in hearing loss may be due to developmental learning disabilities consequent to the exposure to the metal (Schwartz & Otto, 1991; Bellinger, 1995). However, given the current evidence from several human studies, we recommend treating lead as an ototoxic agent.

Mercury (Methyl Mercury Chloride, Mercuric Sulfide)

Occupational exposure to inhaled mercury vapor occurs in many industrial applications, including the production of caustic soda and chlorine, and in the manufacture of thermometers, thermostats, fluorescent light bulbs, batteries, and manometers. Since mercury is known to be neurotoxic, many studies have focused only on the central auditory system, whereas other studies have shown that acute or chronic exposure to mercury generates alterations in both the peripheral and/or central auditory systems (Murata et al., 2004; Rothwell & Boyd, 2008; Prasher, 2009). A recent cross sectional study was carried out by

Al-Betanony et al. (2013) on 138 workers and 151 matched controls in a fluorescent lamp factory in Egypt. The measured noise levels inside the factory were below the maximal permissible limit of the sound intensity inside closed working areas (90 dB according to the Egyptian low). Audiometric air conduction results showed a significantly higher prevalence of hearing loss in the exposed than the comparison group. Other mercury compounds such as dimethyl-mercury, methyl-mercury, and mercuric sulfide have been shown to affect auditory brain stem potentials (Pazderová et al., 1974; Chuu et al., 2001; Clarkson & Magos, 2006).

Cadmium

Industrial use of cadmium mainly occurs in nickel-cadmium batteries, PVC plastics, and paint pigments. Cadmium has a dose-dependent deleterious effect on the auditory system in animal models, causing apoptosis and arrangement alteration of inner ear receptor cells leading to an elevation in auditory thresholds (Ozcaglar et al., 2001; Kim et al., 2008). A probable ototoxic action of cadmium in association with noise exposure was shown by De Abreu & Suzuki (2002), who observed more severe auditory damages, at the frequencies of 4000 and 6000 Hz, in a group of workers exposed to noise and cadmium than in the subjects exposed only to noise.

Chromium

Chromium is used in the manufacturing of stainless steel and to produce several alloys, in plating, corrosion inhibition, wood preservatives, glassware-cleaning solutions, metal finishing and in the production of pigments. In a recent experimental study on animal models, Zhan et al. (2012) found auditory damages with flatness of auditory brain stem responses (ABR) in rats exposed to chromium. Besides, a protective effect of copper and manganese has been supposed, since it has been observed a certain restoration of the hearing function in rats. Regarding human occupational studies, the multiple exposures to a mixture of chromium and lead in combination with noise and their effects on the auditory system were examined by Muttamara & Leong (2004). Elevated concentrations of chromium and lead were found in biological matrices (blood and urine) of exposed workers, as well as high levels of noise, frequently higher than 90 dBA. According to the audiometric test, the workers showed signs of noise-induced hearing loss, but the effect of the co-exposure to the heavy metals cannot be excluded.

Tin

Organic tin compounds are used as heat stabilizers for polyvinyl chloride in piping, siding, and window casings, as antifouling marine paints, wood preservatives fungicides and acaricides. Structural alterations of the auditory system, such as losses or shortening of outer hair cells (OHC) in the basal turn of the cochlea and loss of type 1 spiral ganglion cells, have been reported in animal exposed to trimethyltin (Ruppert et al., 1984; Hoeffding & Fechter,

1991) and triethyltin (Clerici et al., 1993). No study on the effect of occupational exposure to tin compounds on human auditory system has been found in the recent literature.

Arsenic

Arsenic is used in the smelting process of copper, zinc, and lead, as well as in the manufacturing of chemicals and glass. Target organs are: blood, kidneys, and the central nervous, digestive, and skin systems. Animal studies of compounds containing arsenic (sodium arsenilate and its acetylated derivative) have shown histopathological changes in the organ of Corti and the stria vascularis (Anniko, 1976; Miller, 1985). Hearing loss, with particularly marked changes in low-frequency region, has been also reported in human exposed to arsenic pollution (Bencko & Symon, 1977).

To summarize, although some studies show conflicting results, data seem to confirm previous observation of auditory toxicity in workers exposed to lead; and selenium was supposed to reduce its ototoxic effect. Mercury, as well as other compounds containing mercury, affects hearing, with central conduction time delay, but cochlear function may be unaffected. Cadmium causes dose-dependent loss of hearing in animal models; chromium is assumed to worsen the ototoxic action of noise and lead in humans. Studies on arsenic and tin exposures show structural alterations of the auditory system in animal models and low- and high-frequency loss with balance disturbance in humans. Finally, recent studies on cochlear organotypic cultures and animal models (Mao et al., 2011; Apostoli et al., 2013), have confirmed previous findings on the ototoxic properties of other metals, such as manganese and cobalt, which can be also exacerbated by noise exposure.

Table 2. Studies on auditory effects in animals and workers exposed to metals

Substance [CAS]	ACGIH TLV-TWA (STEL)*	Industrial uses	Weight of evidence		References
			Animal models	Human studies	
Lead [7439-92-1]	0.05 mg/m^3	Car batteries, soldering and electrodes in the process of electrolysis, cable covering, plumbing, glazing	O	O /PO	Yamamura et al., 1989; Lasky et al., 1995; Chuang et al., 2007; Hwang, 2009; Galal et al., 2011; Counter et al., 2009
Mercury [7439-97-6]	0.025 mg/m^3	Production of caustic soda and chlorine, manufacture of thermometers, thermostats, fluorescent light bulbs, batteries, and manometers	O	PO	Murata et al., 2004; Rothwell & Boyd, 2008; Prasher, 2009; Al-Betanony et al., 2013
Cadmium [7440-43-9]	0.01 mg/m^3	Nickel-cadmium batteries, PVC plastics, paint pigments	O	PO	Ozcaglar et al., 2001; De Abreu &Suzuki, 2002; Kim et al., 2008
Chromium [7440-47-3]	0.5 mg/m^3	Stainless steel, plating, metal finishing, wood preservative, production of pigments	O/PO	PO	Muttamara & Leong, 2004; Zhan et al., 2012
Tin [7440-31-5]	2 mg/m^3	Stabilizer, antifouling marine plants	PO	NE	Hoeffding & Fechter, 1991; Clerici et al., 1993
Arsenic [7440-38-2]	0.01 mg/m^3	Smelting process, chemicals and glass manufacturing	PO	PO	Anniko, 1976; Miller, 1985

CAS: Chemical Abstracts Service; TLV: Threshold Limit Value – TWA: time-weighted average; STEL: Short-Term Exposure Limit; O: ototoxic substance, PO: possibly ototoxic substance, NC: nonconclusive, NE: no evidence.

Pesticides

Several pesticides are expected to be neurotoxic to humans; consequently these compounds may also affect auditory system. In the following section two classes of potential neurotoxic pesticides are evaluated for their effects on auditory system in exposed workers: organophosphates (OPs) and pyrethroids.

Organophosphates (OPs)

OPs represent the largest class of insecticides sold worldwide. Hoshino et al. (2008) studied associations between hearing impairments and chronic exposure to OPs at low doses on a cohort of 18 Brazilian rural workers. Audiometric tests found that 7 exposed (38.8%) had altered results, 4 of them (22.22%) with decreased performances at high frequencies and the remaining 3 subjects (16.67%) with sensorineural hearing loss. Besides, the authors observed associations between time of exposure and test results. The combined effect of noise and OPs on auditory systems was investigated by Guida et al. (2010). Two groups of 40 individuals each, exposed to malathion and noise (group I) and to noise only (group II) were considered. Both groups showed similar hearing loss values in the high frequencies, but at frequencies of 3 kHz (left ear) and 4 KHz (bilaterally) significant differences were found, with a worsening of thresholds for group I. As the more pronounced hearing loss was found in individuals exposed to both elements, it is conceivable a possible interaction between noise and OPs. Similar findings were observed on 43 rural workers exposed to OPs by Camarinha et al. (2011). A high percentage of subjects (83.7%) resulted with worse than expected responses and the results were consistent for all three tests performed – Frequency Pattern Test (FTP), Duration Pattern Test (DPT) and Gaps-in-noise (GIN) test.

Pyrethroids

Pyrethroids are modern insecticides, in most cases more neurotoxic to insects and less neurotoxic to humans than organophosphates. Two types of pyrethroid structures exist: type II contain a cyano-group in the α-position, whereas type I do not contain a cyano-group (Bradberry et al., 2005). Human pyrethroid poisoning is rare, and almost entirely involves type II. The ototoxic effects of the exposure to a mixture containing pyrethroids and OPs have been investigated by a large study among 14,229 subjects (Crawford et al., 2008). The authors found some evidence that pesticide exposures, including poisoning and medical treatment after high exposure events, could increase the incidence of self-reported hearing loss. In particular, the odds ratio for the highest quartile of exposure was 1.19 (95% CI 1.04-1.35) for insecticides and 1.17 (95% CI 1.04-1.35) for OPs. On the contrary, carbamates, organochlorines and pyrethroids resulted not associated with hearing loss.

In two different studies, published in 2000 and 2004 respectively, Beckett et al. obtained conflicting results. In the first study (Beckett et al., 2000) a statistically significant association ($p<0.05$) was found between hearing loss and pesticide mixture exposure (mainly OPs and pyrethroids) of 185 farm workers. Furthermore, the exposed group presented a higher incidence (3%) of auditory damages compared to controls. Contrary to these previous findings, the authors found no significant association between pesticide exposure and hearing loss in their further 5-year follow-up study (Beckett et al., 2004). Possible biases, such as the smaller sample size (n=65) than the previous study (n=185), the non-random selection of participating subjects, and the exposure estimation based on recall, might have jeopardized the results of this second survey.

The literature linking pesticide exposure to hearing loss is sparse. Results from recent studies suggest that occupational exposure to some pesticides can induce damage to the central auditory system. Nevertheless, no meaningful conclusions can be drawn, also considering a number of deficiencies of some of the examined studies, such as the lack of detailed information on the level of the exposures. No evidence on the potentiation of noise-induced auditory impairments can be supported. Finally, since many pesticide formulations include solvents, metals, and other so-called inert ingredients, it is possible that these exposures can play a role in the association between hearing loss and pesticide exposure.

Other Chemicals

There is growing evidence that other chemicals, such as polychlorinated biphenyls (PCBs) and asphyxiants, produce oxidative stress in the cochlea and consequently may have ototoxic potential by themselves and can potentiate noise-induced hearing loss as well (Fechter et al., 2002a.b, 2003; Morata, 2003; Pouyatos et al., 2005, 2007). Occupational exposure to asphyxiant gases is mainly a result of accidental events; therefore, in this section we will analyze the effects on the auditory system of the only carbon monoxide (CO), for which a chronic occupational exposure cannot be excluded.

Table 3. Epidemiological studies on ototoxic action of occupational exposure to pesticides

Pesticide class	Exposed	Controls	Noise	Auditory test	Weight of evidence	Reference
OPs	n = 18	-	NR	Audiometry, VENG, three questionnaires	PO	Hoshino et al., 2008
	n = 40	n = 40	98.5 dB(A)	Audiometry, interview, acoustic-immittance measures	PO	Guida et al., 2010
	n = 48	-	NR	Audiometry, FTP, DPT and GIN, questionnaire	PO	Camarinha et al., 2011
	n = 18	-	NR	Audiometry, VENG, three questionnaires	PO	Hoshino et al., 2008
Pyrethroids and OPs	65	-	76.4÷93dB(A)	Self-reported interview	NE	Beckett et al., 2004
	n = 4926	n = 9303	YES	Self-reported interview	PO	Crawford et al., 2008

n, number of subjects; NR, not reported; VENG, Vector Electronystagmography; FTP, Frequency Pattern Test; DPT, Duration Pattern Test; GIN, Gaps-in-noise; PO: possibly ototoxic substance, NE: no evidence.

Polychlorinated Biphenyls (PCBs)

Polychlorinated biphenyls (PCBs) consist of 209 synthetic organic compounds, called "congeners," in which 1 to 10 chlorine atoms are attached to a biphenyl ring. Occupational exposure to PCBs can take place during the renovating and demolishing of buildings, repair and maintenance of PCB transformers, accidents, fires, or spills involving PCB transformers and older computers and instruments, and disposal of PCB materials. Rodent studies provided the first evidence for auditory deficits after developmental PCBs exposure. Perinatal exposure to a commercial PCB mixture, Aroclor 1254 (A1254), resulted in long-lasting low-frequency hearing loss (Goldey et al., 1995). The cochlea was specifically indicated as the likely site of action in a study that found loss of outer hair cells in perinatally PCB-exposed rats (Crofton et al., 2000). The effects of developmental exposure to PCBs on cochlear function seem to be confirmed also by cross-sectional epidemiological studies on children (Longnecker et al., 2004; Trnovec et al., 2008; Newman et al., 2009; Boucher et al., 2010). No current occupational studies were identified.

Carbon Monoxide (CO)

CO is generated by incomplete combustion of any carbon-containing fuel or materials in machines or fire accidents. Occupational exposure to CO, often in combination with noise, notably concerns firemen (Treitman et al., 1980; Lees, 1995; Melius, 2001; Fechter et al., 2002), as well as car mechanics, traffic police and parking lot attendants, bus drivers, truck drivers and taxi drivers (Steenland, 1996; Wickramatillake et al., 1998; Morley et al., 1999; Fechter et al., 2002), motor sport athletes (Walker et al., 2001), service stations workers (Kamei & Yanagisawa, 1997; Herbert et al., 2001), industrial cooks. Studies on animal models have demonstrated the ototoxic action of carbon monoxide and the potentiation of noise induced hearing loss by CO. The auditory dysfunction produced by carbon monoxide is frequency-specific, as the basal high frequency region of the cochlea is more vulnerable to its effect (Tawackoli et al., 2001). Over the human auditory system, the negative effects of CO exposure have been described mainly after acute exposures to CO (Mehrparvar et al., 2013; Berent et al., 2005; Razzaq et al., 2010). These studies confirm a potential ototoxic action of CO on human auditory system, but did not control or report exposure to noise as a contributor to the observed hearing deficits. The only recent study on the effect of chronic exposure to low level of carbon monoxide in a noisy work environment has been published by Lacerda et al. (2005). The authors analyzed a database with 8647 hearing exams realized by the Quebec National Institute of Public Health between 1983 and 1996. The results demonstrated significant differences ($p<0.001$) in the auditory thresholds of groups I, composed by subjects exposed to CO and noise (90dBA) and group II, exposed only to noise (90dBA), especially for high frequencies (3, 4 and 6 kHz). These findings in humans and the available evidence on animal models indicate the need for further research on the effects of CO exposure to the auditory system, particularly in populations exposed simultaneously to CO and noise in the workplace (WHO, 1994; Morata et al., 2002).

Conclusion

Recent studies have brought attention to the occupational exposure assessment to ototoxic chemicals. Given the growing complexity of the workplace environment, where various ototoxic agents can be simultaneously present, a clear relationship between chemicals and hearing impairment is difficult to assess with epidemiological studies. Quite often, in fact, workers were exposed to various substances that can interact in a synergistic, additive and sub-additive way, highlighting the need to develop further studies, which can provide a better understanding of the dose-effect relationship. The findings over the literature of the last decade suggest that chemicals such as solvents, metals and pesticides may have ototoxic properties. In particular, human studies in workers exposed to solvents including styrene, toluene, p-xylene, have shown a higher prevalence of hearing loss among solvent-exposed workers when compared with unexposed controls. It is a concern that, in some studies, increased risk of hearing loss was found at exposure concentrations of toluene and styrene lower than the recommended exposure limits. Furthermore, studies carried out in both animal models and human subjects exposed to metals, such as lead, mercury, chromium and cadmium, indicate that these chemicals may result in auditory dysfunction. There are indications that also other organic pollutants, such as pesticides and PCBs, are associated with poorer hearing thresholds of the exposed population, which consists not only of workers but also of particularly vulnerable subjects, such as children and pregnant women.

A concomitant agent very often present in many workplaces is noise exposure. Epidemiological studies report conflicting data, but in some cases indicate a conceivable interaction between chemicals and noise, at least for high exposure levels. No meaningful conclusions, however, can be drawn, also considering a number of uncertainties of these studies, including the lack of detailed information on levels and modalities of the exposure and the deficiency of comparable exposure between groups. Furthermore, in most of these studies, the chronic effects were related to chemical concentrations and noise levels measured at the time of the study, which in some cases could result different than those ascertained in past years. While awaiting more evidence for dose-response assessments, for precautionary action, work exposure standards cannot rule out a likely relationship between solvent exposure and hearing impairments. In conclusion, it is believed useful to report the following recommendations as a general guideline for industrial hygienists:

- Risk management measures aimed at reducing exposure to ototoxic substances should be encouraged.
- For workers co-exposed to noise and ototoxic substances a more frequent health surveillance should be considered, regardless of the level of exposure to noise.
- Appropriate tools should be developed for early diagnosis of chemically induced hearing impairment. Otoacoustic emissions tests could be a valuable complement to pure tone audiometry.
- In workplaces characterized by simultaneous exposure to noise and ototoxic substances, on the basis of the precautionary principle, the use of personal protective equipment by the noise from exposure levels greater than 80 dB (A) should be recommended.

- Finally, training and information of workers should highlight the risk of possible synergistic effect of exposure to chemicals ototoxic and noise.

References

Al-Batanony, M.A.; Abdel-Rasul, G.M.; Abu-Salem, M.A; Al-Dalatony M.M.; Allam, H.K. (2013). Occupational exposure to mercury among workers in a fluorescent lamp factory, Quisna industrial zone, *Egypt. Int. J. Occup. Environ. Med.,* 4, 149-156.

Albee, R.R.; Spencer, P.J.; Johnson, K.A.; Bradley, G.J.; Marable, B.R.; Wilmer, J.W.; Mattsson, J.L. (2006). Lack of trigeminal nerve toxicity in rats exposed to trichloroethylene vapor for 13 weeks. *Int. J. Toxicol.,* 25, 531-540.

Anniko, M. (1976). The cytochochleogram in atoxyl-treated guinea pigs. *Acta Otolaryngol.,* 82 (1-2), 70-81.

Apostoli, P.; Catalani, S.; Zaghini, A.; Mariotti, A.; Poliani, P.L.; Vielmi, V.; Semeraro, F.; Duse, S.; Porzionato, A.; Macchi, V.; Padovani, A.; Rizzetti, M.C.; De Caro, R. (2013). High doses of cobalt induce optic and auditory neuropathy. *Exp. Toxicol. Pathol.,* 65 (6), 719-727.

Beckett, W.S.; Chamberlain, D.; Hallman, E.; May, J.; Hwang, S.A.; Gomez, M.; Eberly, S.; Cox, C.; Stark, A. (2000). Hearing conservation for farmers: source apportionment of occupational and environmental factors contributing to hearing loss. *J. Occup. Environ. Med.,* 42, 806- 813.

Beckett, W.S.; Hallman, E.; May, J.; Hwang, S.A.; Gomez, M.; Eberly, S.; Cox, C. (2004). Follow-up to farm family health and hazard survey. *J. Occup. Environ. Med.,* 46, 314-315.

Bellinger, D.C. (1995). Interpreting the literature on lead and child development: the neglected role of the "experimental system". *Neurotoxicol. Teratol.*, 17, 201-212.

Bencko, V.; Symon. K. (1977). Test of environmental exposure to arsenic and hearing changes in exposed children. *Environ. Health Perspect.,* 19, 95–101.

Berent, A.C.; Todd, J.; Sergeeff, J.; Powell, L.L. (2005). Carbon monoxide toxicity: A case series. *J. Vet. Emerg. Crit. Care,* 15 (2), 128-135.

Bonfiglioli, R.; Carnevali, L.; Di Lello, M.; Violante, F.S. (2014). Bilateral hearing loss after dichloromethane poisoning: A case report. *Am. J. Ind. Med.,* 57 (2), 254-257.

Boucher, O.; Bastien, C.H.; Saint-Amour, D.; Dewailly, T.; Ayotte, P.; Jacobson, J.L.; Muckle, G. (2010). Prenatal exposure to methylmercury and PCBs affects distinct stages of information processing: An event-related potential study with inuit children. *Neurotoxicology,* 31 (4), 373-384.

Bradberry, S.M.; Cage, S.A.; Proudfoot, A.T.; Vale, J.A. (2005). Poisoning due to pyrethroids. *Toxicol. Rev.,* 24, 93-106.

Camarinha, C.R.; Frota, S.M.; Pacheco-Ferreira, H.; Lima, M.A. (2011). Auditory temporal processing assessment in rural workers exposed to organophosphate pesticides. *J. Soc. Bras. Fonoaudiol.,* 23 (2), 102-106.

Campo, P.; Lataye, R.; Loquet, G.; Bonnet, P. (2001). Styrene-induced hearing loss: a membrane insult, *Hear. Res.,* 154, 170-180.

Cappaert, N.L.; Klis, S.F.; Baretta, A.B.; Muijser, H.; Smoorenburg, G.F. (2000). Ethyl benzene-induced ototoxicity in rats: a dose-dependent mid-frequency hearing loss. *J. Assoc. Res. Otolaryngol.,* 1, 292-299.

Cappaert, N.L.; Klis, S.F.; Muijser, H.; de Groot, J.C.; Kulig, B.M.; Smoorenburg, G.F. (1999). The ototoxic effects of ethyl benzene in rats', *Hear. Res.,* 137 (1-2), 91-102.

Chang, S.J.; Shih, T.S.; Chou, T.C.; Chen, C.J.; Chang, H.Y.; Sung, F.C. (2003). Hearing loss in workers exposed to carbon disulfide and noise. Environ. *Health. Perspect.,111,*1620-1624.

Chang, S.J.; Chen, C.J.; Lien, C.H.; Sung, F.C. (2006). Hearing loss in workers exposed to toluene and noise. *Environ. Health. Perspect.,* 114,1283-1286.

Choi, S.W.; Peek-Asa, C.; Sprince, N.L.; Rautiainen, R.H.; Donham, K.J.; Flamme, G.A.; Whitten, P.S.; Zwerling, C. (2005). Hearing loss as a risk factor for agricultural injuries. *Am. J. Ind. Med.,* 48 (4), 293-301.

Choi, Y.H.; Hu, H.; Mukherjee, B.; Miller, J.; Park, S.K. (2012). Environmental cadmium and lead exposures and hearing loss in U.S. adults: the National Health and Nutrition Examination Survey, 1999 to 2004. *Environ. Health Perspect., 120* (11), 1544-1550.

Chuu, J.J.; Hsu, C.J.; Lin-Shiau, S.Y. (2001). Abnormal auditory brainstem responses for mice treated with mercurial compounds: involvement of excessive nitric oxide. *Toxicology,* 162 (1), 11-22.

Clarkson, T.W.; Magos, L. (2006). The toxicology of mercury and its chemical compounds. *Crit. Rev. Toxicol.,* 36 (8), 609-662.

Clerici, W.J.; Chertoff, M.E.; Brownell, W.E.; Fechter, L.D. (1993). In vitro organotin administration alters guinea pig cochlear outer hair cell shape and viability. *Toxicol. Appl. Pharmacol.,* 120 (2), 193-202.

Counter, S.A.; Buchanan, L.H.; Ortega, F. (2009). Neurophysiologic and neurocognitive case profiles of Andean patients with chronic environmental lead poisoning. *J. Toxicol. Environ. Health* A, 72 (19), 1150-1159.

Crawford, J.M.; Hoppin, J.A.; Alavanja, M.C.; Blair, A.; Sandler, D.P.; Kamel, F. (2008). Hearing loss among licensed pesticide applicators in the agricultural health study. *J. Occup. Environ. Med.,* 50 (7), 817-826.

de Abreu, M.T.; Suzuki, F.A. (2002) Audiometric evaluation of workers exposed to noise and cadmium. *Rev. Bras. Otorinolaringol,* 68 (4), 488-494.

Draper, T.H.J.; Bamiou, D.E. (2009). Auditory neuropathy in a patient exposed to xylene: case report. *J. Laryngol. Otol.,* 123, 462-465.

Fechter, L.D.; Chen, G.D.; Rao, D. (2002a). Chemical Asphyxiants and Noise. *Noise Health.,* 4 (14), 49-61.

Fechter, L.D.; Chen, G.D.; Johnson, D.L. (2002b). Potentiation of noise-induced hearing loss by low concentrations of hydrogen cyanide in rats. *Toxicol. Sci.,* 66 (1), 131-138.

Fechter, L.D.; Klis, S.F.; Shirwany, N.A.; Moore, T.G.; Rao, D.B. (2003). Acrylonitrile produces transient cochlear function loss and potentiates permanent noise-induced hearing loss. *Toxicol.Sci.,* 75 (1), 117-123.

Fuente, A.; McPherson, B. (2007). Central auditory processing effects induced by solvent exposure. *Int.J.Occup.Med.Environ.Health,* 20 (3), 271-279.

Fuente, A.; McPherson, B.; Cardemil, F. (2013). Xylene-induced auditory dysfunction in humans. *Ear Hear.,* 34 (5), 651-660.

Fuente, A.; McPherson, B.; Hickson, L. (2011). Central auditory dysfunction associated with exposure to a mixture of solvents. *Int.J.Audiol.,* 50 (12), 857-865.

Gagnaire, F.; Langlais, C. (2005). Relative ototoxicity of 21 aromatic solvents. *Arch.Toxicol.,* 79 (6), 346-354.

Gagnaire, F.; Marignac, B.; Langlais, C.; Bonnet, P. (2001). Ototoxicity in rats exposed to ortho-, meta- and para-xylene vapours for 13 weeks. *Pharmacol.Toxicol.,* 89 (1), 6-14.

Galal, S.; El-Samra, G.H.; Mazhar, M.; El-Kholy, F.; Hegazy, A. (2011). Risk Behaviour of lead-exposed Workers and Hearing Impairment. *Int. J. Collab. Res. Internal Med. Public Health,* 3 (2), 132-142.

Gatto, M.P.; Fioretti, M.; Fabrizi, G.; Gherardi, M.; Strafella, E.; Santarelli, L. (2014). Effects of potential neurotoxic pesticides on hearing loss: a review. *Neurotoxicology,* 42 , 24-32.

Gelbke, H.P.; Goen, T.; Maurer, M.; Sulsky, S.I. (2009). A review of health effects of carbon disulfide in viscose industry and a proposal for an occupational exposure limit. *Crit.Rev.Toxicol.,* 39 Suppl 2 , 1-126.

Goldey, E.S.; Kehn, L.S.; Lau, C.; Rehnberg, G.L.; Crofton, K.M. (1995). Developmental exposure to polychlorinated biphenyls (Aroclor 1254) reduces circulating thyroid hormone concentrations and causes hearing deficits in rats. *Toxicol.Appl.Pharmacol.,* 135 (1), 77-88.

Guida, H.L.; Morini, R.G.; Cardoso, A.C. (2010). Audiological evaluation in workers exposed to noise and pesticide. *Braz J.Otorhinolaryngol.,* 76 (4), 423-427.

Herbert, R.; Szeinuk, J.; O'brien, S. (2001).Occupational health problems of bridge and tunnel officers. *Occup. Med-State Art,* 16 (1), 51-65.

Hetu, R.; Getty, L.; Quoc, H.T. (1995). Impact of occupational hearing loss on the lives of workers. *Occup. Med.,* 10 (3), 495-512.

Hoeffding, V.; Fechter, L.D. (1991). Trimethyltin disrupts auditory function and cochlear morphology in pigmented rats. *Neurotoxicol. Teratol.,* 13 (2), 135-145.

Hoffmann, J.; Ihrig, A.; Hoth, S.; Triebig, G. (2006). Field study to explore possible effects of styrene on auditory function in exposed workers. *Ind. Health,* 44 (2), 283-286.

Hoshino, A.C.; Pacheco-Ferreira, H.; Taguchi, C.K.; Tomita, S.; Miranda Mde, F. (2008). Ototoxicity study in workers exposed to organophosphate. *Braz. J. Otorhinolaryngol.,* 74 (6), 912-918.

Hwang, S.A.; Gomez, M.I.; Sobotova, L.; Stark, A.D.; May, J.J.; Hallman, E.M. (2001). Predictors of hearing loss in New York farmers. *Am. J. Ind. Med.,* 40 (1), 23-31.

Johnson, A.C.; Juntunen, L.; Nylen, P.; Borg, E.; Hoglund, G. (1988). Effect of interaction between noise and toluene on auditory function in the rat. *Acta Otolaryngol.,* 105 (1-2), 56-63.

Johnson, A.C.; Morata, T.C.; Lindblad, A.C.; Nylen, P.R.; Svensson, E.B.; Krieg, E.; Aksentijevic, A.; Prasher, D. (2006). Audiological findings in workers exposed to styrene alone or in concert with noise. *Noise Health.,* 8 (30), 45-57.

Jones, L.G.; Prins, J.; Park, S.; Walton, J.P.; Luebke, A.E.; Lurie, D.I. (2008). Lead exposure during development results in increased neurofilament phosphorylation, neuritic beading, and temporal processing deficits within the murine auditory brainstem. *J. Comp. Neurol.,* 506 (6), 1003-1017.

Kamei, M.; Yanagisawa, Y. (1997). Estimation of CO exposure of road construction workers in tunnel. *Ind. Health,* 35 (1), 119-125.

Kaufman, L.R.; LeMasters, G.K.; Olsen, D.M.; Succop, P. (2005). Effects of concurrent noise and jet fuel exposure on hearing loss. *J. Occup. Environ. Med.,* 47 (3), 212-218.

Kim, J.; Park, H.; Ha, E.; Jung, T.; Paik, N.; Yang, S. (2005). Combined effects of noise and mixed solvents exposure on the hearing function among workers in the aviation industry. *Ind. Health,* 43 (3), 567-573.

Kim, S.J.; Jeong, H.J.; Myung, N.Y.; Kim, M.C.; Lee, J.H.; So, H.S.; Park, R.K.; Kim, H.M.; Um, J.Y.; Hong, S.H. (2008). The protective mechanism of antioxidants in cadmium-induced ototoxicity in vitro and in vivo. *Environ. Health Perspect., 116* (7), 854-862.

Lacerda, A.; Leroux, T.; Gagn, J.P. (2005). The combined effect of noise and carbon monoxide on hearing thresholds of exposed workers. *J. Acoust. Soc. Am., 1*17 (4), 2481-2481.

Lasky, R.E.; Maier, M.M.; Snodgrass, E.B.; Hecox, K.E.; Laughlin, N.K. (1995). The effects of lead on otoacoustic emissions and auditory evoked potentials in monkeys. *Neurotoxicol. Teratol.,* 17 (6), 633-644.

Lees, P.S. (1995). Combustion products and other firefighter exposures. *Occup. Med.,* 10 (4), 691-706.

Li, H.S.; Johnson, A.C.; Borg, E.; Hoglund, G. (1992). Auditory degeneration after exposure to toluene in two genotypes of mice. *Arch. Toxicol.,* 66 (6), 382-386.

Maguin, K.; Lataye, R.; Campo, P.; Cossec, B.; Burgart, M.; Waniusiow, D. (2006). Ototoxicity of the three xylene isomers in the rat. *Neurotoxicol. Teratol.,* 28 (6), 648-656.

Mao, X.; Wong, A.A.; Crawford, R.W. (2011). Cobalt toxicity--an emerging clinical problem in patients with metal-on-metal hip prostheses? *Med. J. Aust.,* 194 (12), 649-651.

Mascagni, P.; Formenti, C.; Pettazzoni, M.; Feltrin, G.; Toffoletto, F. (2007). Hearing function and solvent exposure: study of a worker population exposed to styrene. *G. Ital. Med. Lav. Ergon.,* 29 (3 Suppl), 277-279.

Mehrparvar, A.H.; Davari, M.H.; Mollasadeghi, A.; Vahidi, M.R.; Mostaghaci, M.; Bahaloo, M.; Shokouh, P. (2013). Hearing Loss due to Carbon Monoxide Poisoning. *Case Rep. Otolaryngol.,* 2013 , 940187.

Melius, J. (2001). Occupational health for firefighters. *Occup. Med.,* 16 (1), 101-108.

Miller, J.J. (1985*). Handbook of ototoxicity,* CRC Press, Boca Raton.

Morata, T.C. (2003). Chemical exposure as a risk factor for hearing loss. *J. Occup. Environ. Med.,* 45 (7), 676-682.

Morata, T.C. (1989). Study of the effects of simultaneous exposure to noise and carbon disulfide on workers' hearing. *Scand. Audiol.,* 18 (1), 53-58.

Morata, T.C.; Dunn, D.E.; Sieber, W.K. (1994). Occupational exposure to noise and ototoxic organic solvents. *Arch. Environ. Health,* 49, 359–365.

Morata, T.C.; Johnson, A.C.; Nylen, P.; Svensson, E.B.; Cheng, J.; Krieg, E.F.; Lindblad, A.C.; Ernstgard, L.; Franks, J. (2002). Audiometric findings in workers exposed to low levels of styrene and noise. *J. Occup. Environ. Med.,* 44 (9), 806-814.

Morata, T.C.; Sliwinska-Kowalska, M.; Johnson, A.C.; Starck, J.; Pawlas, K.; Zamyslowska-Szmytke, E.; Nylen, P.; Toppila, E.; Krieg, E.; Pawlas, N.; Prasher, D. (2011). A multicenter study on the audiometric findings of styrene-exposed workers. *Int. J. Audiol.,* 50 (10), 652-660.

Morioka, I.; Kuroda, M.; Miyashita, K.; Takeda, S. (1999). Evaluation of organic solvent ototoxicity by the upper limit of hearing. *Arch. Environ. Health,* 54 (5), 341–346.

Morley, J.C.; Seitz, T.; Tubbs, R. (1999). Carbon monoxide and noise exposure at a monster truch and motocross show. *Appl. Occup. Environ. Hyg.,* 14 (10), 645-655.

Muijser, H.; Hoogendijk, E.M.; Hooisma, J. (1988). The effects of occupational exposure to styrene on high-frequency hearing thresholds. *Toxicology,* 49 (2-3), 331-340.

Murata, K.; Weihe, P.; Budtz-Jorgensen, E.; Jorgensen, P.J.; Grandjean, P. (2004). Delayed brainstem auditory evoked potential latencies in 14-year-old children exposed to methylmercury. *J. Pediatr.,* 144 (2), 177-183.

Muttamara, S; Leong, S.T. (2004). Health implication among occupational exposed workers in a chromium alloy factory, Thailand. *J. Environ. Sci.* (China),16 (2),181-186.

Newman, J.; Gallo, M.V.; Schell, L.M.; DeCaprio, A.P.; Denham, M.; Deane, G.D.; Akwesasne Task Force on Environment (2009). Analysis of PCB congeners related to cognitive functioning in adolescents. *Neurotoxicology,* 30 (4), 686-696.

Nylen, P.; Hagman, M.; Johnson, A.C. (1994). Function of the auditory and visual systems, and of peripheral nerve, in rats after long-term combined exposure to n-hexane and methylated benzene derivatives. I. Toluene. *Pharmacol. Toxicol.,* 74 (2), 116-123.

Ozcaglar, H.U.; Agirdir, B.; Dinc, O.; Turhan, M.; Kilincarslan, S.; Oner, G. (2001). Effects of cadmium on the hearing system. *Acta Otolaryngol.,* 121 (3), 393-397.

Pazderova, J.; Jirasek, A.; Mraz, M.; Pechan, J. (1974). Post-mortem findings and clinical signs of dimethyl mercury poisoning in man. *Int. Arch. Arbeitsmed.,* 33 (4), 323-328.

Pouyatos, B.; Gearhart, C.A.; Fechter, L.D. (2005). Acrylonitrile potentiates hearing loss and cochlear damage induced by moderate noise exposure in rats. *Toxicol. Appl. Pharm.,* 204 (1); 46-56.

Pouyatos, B.; Gearhart, C.; Nelson-Miller, A.; Fulton, S.; Fechter, L. (2007). Oxidative stress pathways in the potentiation of noise-induced hearing loss by acrylonitrile. *Hear. Res.,* 224 (1-2), 61-74.

Prasher, D. (2009). Heavy metals and noise exposure: Health effects. *Noise Health,* 11 (44), 141-144.

Prasher, D.; Morata, T; Campo, P.; Fechter, L.; Johnson, A.C.; Lund, S.P., Pawlas, K., Starck, J., Sliwinska-Kowalska, M.; Sulkowski, W. (2002). NoiseChem : An European Commission research project on the effects of exposure to noise and industrial chemicals on hearing and balance. *Noise Health,* 4, 41-48.

Pryor, G.T.; Howd, R.A. (1986). Toluene-induced ototoxicity by subcutaneous administration. *Neurobeh. Toxicol. Ter.,* 8, 103–104.

Pryor, G.T.; Rebert, C.S.; Howd, R.A. (1987). Hearing loss in rats caused by inhalation of mixed xylenes and styrene. *J. Appl. Toxicol.* 7 (1), 55-61.

Razzaq, M.; Dumbala, S.; Moudgil, S.S. (2010). Sudden deafness due to carbon monoxide poisoning. *J. Neurol. Neurosur. Ps.,* 81 (6), 658.

Rothwell, J.A.; Boyd, P.J. (2008). Amalgam dental fillings and hearing loss. *Int. J. Audiol.,* 47 (12), 770-776.

Ruppert, P.H.; Dean, K.F.; Reiter, L.W. (1984). Trimethyltin disrupts acoustic startle responding in adult rats. *Toxicol. Lett.,* 22 (1), 33-38.

Ryback, L.P. (1992). Hearing: The effects of chemicals. Otolaryngol. *Head Neck Surg.,* 106, 677-686.

Saunders, J.E.; Jastrzembski, B.G.; Buckey, J.C.; Enriquez, D.; MacKenzie, T.A.; Karagas, M.R. (2013). Hearing loss and heavy metal toxicity in a Nicaraguan mining community: audiological results and case reports. *Audiol. Neurootol.,* 18 (2),101-113.

Schaper, M.; Demes, P.; Zupanic, M.; Blaszkewicz, M.; Seeber, A. (2003). Occupational toluene exposure and auditory function: results from a follow-up study. *Ann. Occup. Hyg.,* 47 (6), 493-502.

Schwartz, J.; Otto, D. (1991). Lead and minor hearing impairment. *Arch. Environ. Health,* 46 (5), 300-305.

Shargorodsky, J.; Curhan, S.G.; Henderson, E.; Eavey, R.; Curhan, G.C. (2011). Heavy metals exposure and hearing loss in US adolescents. Arch. Otolaryngol. *Head Neck Surg.,* 137 (12), 1183-1189.

Simonsen, L.; Lund, S.P. (1995). Four weeks inhalation exposure to n-heptane causes loss of auditory sensitivity in rats. *Pharmacol. Toxicol.,* 76 (1), 41-46.

Sisto, R.; Cerini, L.; Gatto, M.P.; Gherardi, M.; Gordiani, A.; Sanjust, F.; Paci, E.; Tranfo, G.; Moleti, A. (2013). Otoacoustic emission sensitivity to exposure to styrene and noise. *J. Acoust. Soc. Am.,* 134 (5), 3739-3748.

Sliwińska-Kowalska, M.; Zamyslowska-Szmytke, E.; Szymczak, W.; Kotylo, P.; Fiszer, M.; Wesolowski, W.; Pawlaczyk-Luszczynska, M. (2003). Ototoxic effects of occupational exposure to styrene and co-exposure to styrene and noise. *J. Occup. Environ. Med.,* 45 (1), 15-24.

Sliwinska-Kowalska, M.; Zamyslowska-Szmytke, E.; Szymczak, W.; Kotylo, P.; Fiszer, M.; Wesolowski, W.; Pawlaczyk-Luszczynska, M.; Bak, M.; Gajda-Szadkowska, A. (2004). Effects of coexposure to noise and mixture of organic solvents on hearing in dockyard workers. *J. Occup. Environ. Med.,* 46 (1), 30-38.

Sliwinska-Kowalska, M.; Zamyslowska-Szmytke, E.; Szymczak, W.; Kotylo, P.; Fiszer, M.; Wesolowski, W.; Pawlaczyk-Luszczynska, M. (2005). Exacerbation of noise-induced hearing loss by co-exposure to workplace chemicals. *Environ. Toxicol. Phar.,* 19(3), 547-553.

Sprince, N.L.; Zwerling, C.; Lynch, C.F.; Whitten, P.S.; Thu, K.; Logsden-Sackett, N.; Burmeister, L.F.; Sandler, D.P.; Alavanja, M.C. (2003). Risk factors for agricultural injury: a casecontrol analysis of Iowa farmers in the Agricultural Health Study. *J. Agric. Safety Health,* 9, 5–18.

Steenland, K. (1996). Epidemiology of occupation and coronary heart disease: research agenda. *Am. J. Ind. Med.,* 30 (4), 495-499.

Sullivan, M.J.; Rarey, K.E.; Conolly, R.B. (1988). Ototoxicity of toluene in rats. *Neurotoxicol. Teratol.,* 10 (6), 525-530.

Tawackoli, W.; Chen, G.D.; Fechter, L.D. (2001). Disruption of cochlear potentials by chemical asphyxiants. Cyanide and carbon monoxide. *Neurotoxicol. Teratol.,* 23 (2), 157-165.

Treitman, R.D.; Burgess, W.A.; Gold, A. (1980). Air contaminants encountered by firefighters. *Am. Ind. Hyg. Assoc. J.,* 41 (11), 796-802.

Triebig, G.; Bruckner, T.; Seeber, A. (2009). Occupational styrene exposure and hearing loss: a cohort study with repeated measurements. *Int. Arch. Occup. Environ. Health,* 82 (4), 463-480.

Trnovec, T.; Sovcikova, E.; Hust'ak, M.; Wimmerova, S.; Kocan, A.; Jureckova, D.; Langer, P.; Palkovicova, L.; Drobna, B. (2008). Exposure to polychlorinated biphenyls and hearing impairment in children. *Environ. Toxicol. Pharmacol.,* 25 (2), 183-187.

Vyskocil, A.; Leroux, T.; Truchon, G.; Gendron, M.; El Majidi, N.; Viau, C. (2008a). Occupational ototoxicity of n-hexane. *Hum. Exp. Toxicol.,* 27 (6), 471-476.

Vyskocil, A.; Leroux, T.; Truchon, G.; Lemay, F.; Gagnon, F.; Gendron, M.; Viau, C. (2008b). Ototoxicity of trichloroethylene in concentrations relevant for the working environment. *Hum. Exp. Toxicol.,* 27 (3), 195-200.

Walker, S.M.; Ackland, T.R.; Dawson, B. (2001). The combined effect of heat and carbon monoxide on the performance of motorsport athletes. *Comp. Biochem. Physiol. A. Mol. Integr. Physiol.,* 128 (4), 709 718.

WORLD HEALTH ORGANIZATION - WHO. (1994). International workshop: setting priorities in environmental epidemiology- report on a Word Health Organization Meeting. *Arch. Environ. Health,* 49 (4), 239-245.

Wickramatillake, H.D.; Gun, R.T.; Ryan, P. (1998). Carbon monoxide exposures in Australian workplaces could precipitate myocardial ischaemia in smoking workers with coronary artery disease. *Aust. N. Z. J. Public Health,* 22 (3 Suppl), 389-393.

Yamamura, K.; Terayama, K.; Yamamoto, N.; Kohyama, A.; Kishi, R. (1989). Effects of acute lead acetate exposure on adult guinea pigs: electrophysiological study of the inner ear. *Fundam. Appl. Toxicol.,* 13 (3), 509-515.

Zhan, K.; Wu, S.; Ji, X.; Li, N.; Yu, J.; Gao, X. (2012). Chromium-induced hearing loss in rats and the protective effect of copper and manganese. *Trace Elem. Electroly.,* 29 (1), 72-77.

In: Handbook of Hearing Disorders Research
Editor: Charlotte Hailee Atkinson
ISBN: 978-1-63463-654-4

Chapter 3

Sudden Sensorineural Hearing Loss and Polymorphisms in Iron Homeostasis Genes

D. Gemmati[1], A. Castiglione[2], M. Vigliano[1], A. Ciorba[3] and C. Aimoni[3]
[1]Ctr. Hemostasis & Thrombosis, Dept. of Medical Sciences, University Hospital of Ferrara, Italy
[2]ENT & Otosurgery Department, University Hospital of Padua, Italy
[3]ENT & Audiology Department, University Hospital of Ferrara, Italy

Abstract

Sudden sensorineural hearing loss (SSNHL) is an important cause of acquired hearing deficits in the adults. Several pathophysiological hypothesis have been proposed so far, however the cause of sudden hearing loss is still unclear. Even if local hypoxic/ischemic events as well as inner ear viral infection have been reported to be the main hypothesis leading to transient or permanent cochlear dysfunction, and therefore to Sudden Sensorineural Hearing Loss, still there are other hypothesis that have been claimed.

Aim of the present study is to investigate about the possible role of iron metabolism, and in particular about the presence of genetic variants of the principal iron-related genes, and acute inner ear disorders such as sudden sensorineural hearing loss.

Introduction

Sudden sensorineural hearing loss (SSNHL) represents an acute inner ear disorder, mostly unilateral, that generally affect adults worldwide, even if higher occurrence rates are reported in developed countries [1, 2]. It has been estimated that SSNHL has an overall incidence rate of 5–20 / 100,000 individuals per year, though this is most likely an underestimate [2, 3].

Several pathophysiological mechanisms for idiopathic SSNHL have been proposed in the literature. The most reported are: local hypoxic/ischemic events (such as coagulopathies, vascular hypotension and thrombo-embolism), autoimmune disorders, metabolic diseases, viral inner ear infections, rupture of the inner ear membranes, free radicals induced-damage, neuronal damage and dysregulation of the local inflammatory response [3-5] leading to transient or permanent dysfunction of cochlear microcirculation [6].

Since iron has been linked to oxidative stress, we hypothesized that iron metabolism regulatory genes could have a role in the homeostasis of the oxidative balance also in the inner ear and, consequently, in the pathophysiology of acute inner ear disorders such as SSNHL.

Aim of this chapter is to focus on the possible role of divalent metallic ions, and in particular on the presence of genetic variants of the principal iron-related genes, in the aetiopathogenesis of SSNHL [7].

Methods

The Pubmed database was searched up to September 2014 (going back for 10 years); full text articles were obtained when the title, abstract or key words suggested that the study may be eligible for this study. The search was carried out independently, and restricted to papers in English language. Other papers were also identified from the references in the published literature.

The medical subject heading (MeSH) used included: Sudden Sensorineural Hearing Loss, Iron metabolism, Iron Homeostasis, Iron genes, Oxidative stress, Inner ear.

Iron Metabolism and Oxidative Stress

There is a growing interest in the possible association between iron metabolism and oxidative stress, as it has been reported that local iron excess is a potential cause of increased oxidative stress and therefore could be involved in cellular injury and death. Iron is an essential nutrient, but its divalent form (Fe2+), as well as other divalent metal ions, also retains the capacity to enhance redox cycling and free radical formation [8, 9]. Iron-mediated oxidative stress is hypothesized to be involved in the pathogenesis of several degenerative disorders, including thrombosis, venous ulcers, chronic venous disease, and central nervous system disorders such as multiple sclerosis and other neurodegenerative diseases, or neoplasms [10-13]. In addition, a novel iron-driven aetiopathogenetic mechanism, responsible for increase free radical generation, has been formulated in degenerative skin lesions appearance comprehending coexistence of local iron overload and iron homeostasis gene variants [14]. Similar conditions could also be potentially associated with sudden hearing loss [15]. So, divalent ions homeostasis could be a central pathway involved in the pathophysiology of sudden hearing loss [16, 17, 18].

The main genes and their variants that could be possibly involved in the aetiopathogenesis of SSNHL are described below [10, 19].

The *HFE gene* (6p21.3-22.2) encodes a membrane protein of 348 amino acids that belongs to the MHC class I family. The protein is normally expressed in cryptal enterocytes of the duodenum, liver, placenta, kidney, central nervous system, plasma and platelets. By complexing with beta 2 microglobulin and transferrin receptor 2 (TFR2), it plays a crucial role in iron homeostasis, and, when mutated, it is believed to be responsible for hemochromatosis, variegate porphyria and microvascular complications of diabetes. Gene variants and/or mutated proteins bind to the transferrin receptor and reduce its affinity for iron-loaded transferrin. Thus, they finally unbalance the iron intake. Recent increasing interest in neuro-degenerative disorders mediated by iron overload, have highlighted the HFE gene among candidates for further investigations into iron homeostasis involvement in similar conditions. A review of the literature suggests a potential role even in iron-mediated hearing loss also in the past [20, 21]. Finally, it is important to note that the HFE gene is also expressed in the brain, spinal cord, cortex and cerebellum [22, 23]. Thus, it could be directly involved or responsible for specific conditions concerning the central nervous system.

The *FPN1 (SLC40A1) gene* is located on chromosome 2 (2q32.2), and it encodes a protein (ferroportin) of 570 amino acids with the specific function of exporting iron out from cells in the basolateral space, except for the reticulo-endothelial cells, which can spread iron ions into the blood circulation. Consequently, FPN1 plays a crucial role in iron homeostasis [24], and, generally, it has the opposite function of the divalent metal transporter 1 (DMT1) protein product [25], which allows intracellular passage of divalent iron (Fe2+). Ferroportin is expressed in different tissues, brain and spinal cord included, though to the best of our knowledge, there are no previous reported studies that document its localization specifically into the cochlea. Similar to other iron genes, it undergoes iron regulation at the transcriptional and translational level [26-28].

Another important gene related to ferroportin expression and function is the *HEPC gene (19q13.1)* encoding the protein Hepcidin Anti Microbial Peptide (HAMP). This protein is a 25-amino acid peptide, derived from the cleavage of an 84-amino-acid long pro-peptide that is mainly synthesized by hepatocytes, but it is expressed also in brain, spinal cord, cortex and cerebellum included. HEPC is the major regulator of iron balance activity via binding to the FPN1 protein on the cell membrane, sup-pressing it [29, 30]. HEPC expression and its role in iron homeostasis may play a crucial role in different conditions [31].

The *TF gene (*3q22.1*)* encodes for the protein transferrin, which forms a stable complex with the HFE protein, which facilitates iron transfer via the transferrin receptor. The function of this protein is to transport iron from the intestine, reticuloendothelial system, and liver parenchymal cells to all proliferating cells in the body. Tansferrin is expressed in different tissues, brain, spinal cord included, cortex and cerebellum included. The effect of HFE on iron absorption depends on its relationship with the transferrin receptor. HFE variants affect TF binding, determining a loss of HFE-repressor function for TF uptake, thereby increasing iron transport within the cells [32-34].

Iron Metabolism and the Inner Ear

Sudden hearing loss has been reported to be associated with a huge number of clinical conditions and its aetiopathogenesis is still unclear [35-38]. The uncertainty of reasonable etiologies has encouraged continuous investigations aimed at identifying the most convincing pathological explanations. Far from the identification of an unequivocal mutated gene, the study of genetic variants of several conditions has attracted several researchers even if a specific correlation between a precise inner ear gene mutation and SSNHL still has to be proved. Some studies have reported a correlation of various polymorphisms with an increased [39-43] or reduced [44] risk of developing hearing impairment.

Recent findings concerning ROS-mediated damage, NO activity and inner ear iron metabolism have encouraged researchers to focus their studies on possible connections between microvascular damage and free radical production in the inner ear [45-47, 49]. In this sense, some have speculated that polymorphisms of genes related to iron metabolism, such as FPN1 (SLC40A1) gene, the HFE gene or the TF gene, could be involved in the pathogenesis of some acute inner ear disorders, such as sudden sensorineural hearing loss [47,48,49]. Of particular interesting are the observations among iron metabolism within the stria vascularis. Stria vascularis is particular sensitive to free radical stress due to its high metabolic activity and dense vascular system [50], and, consequently, when iron cheletor proteins are not adequately functioning to contrast and neutralize the damaging effect of iron and linked free radicals, its function can be dramatically impaired, therefore hampering inner ear homeostasis [50]. The significant presence of ferritin [47] and DMT1 [48,49], within the cochlear stria, suggest that these proteins have an active role in restoration and deposition of iron, and can retain a role in reducing the endolymphatic concentration of divalent ions [51, 52]. In fact, preliminary experimental studies on mouse models have shown that free radical stress, induced by the loss of specific protein expression related to iron metabolism in stria vascularis, cause hearing loss [18]. It is possible to speculate that polymorphism of genes related to iron metabolism such as FPN1 (SLC40A1) gene, or of the HFE gene or the TF gene, could possibly contribute in altering the inner ear oxidative homeostasis.

Apart from the stria vascularis, the exact location of the proteins involved in the metabolism of iron, within other inner ear settings, is still not clear. The identification of their position could offer indications in understanding how iron metabolism works within the inner ear oxidative homeostasis.

Unfortunately, the knowledge among the iron metabolism within the inner ear is still very limited; further experimental studies are necessary in order to understand which could be its role within the inner ear homeostasis.

Iron Metabolism and Sudden Sensorineural Hearing Loss

So far, there are no clinical evidences to support this association, clinically. Only very few studies have claimed a relationship between these two conditions. In particular, Chung et al have observed a relation between SSNHL and iron deficiency anemia [53]. Also, Sun et al described significant improvements in clinical results using iron therapy in patients with

SSNHL [54]. However, their clinical success only warranted the use of iron therapy in managing SSNHL, and their limited case numbers meant that the relationship between patients affected by iron deficiency anemia and SSNHL should still be further elucidated [54].

Even if the few available studies on animal models seem to encourage this hypothesis as described in the previous paragraph, the aetiopathogenetic mechanism that links the onset of an acute inner ear disorder, such as SSNHL, and iron metabolism is still far to be understood, though it can be an intriguing hypothesis.

Conclusion

In conclusion, clinical and genetic studies are required to further elucidate the pathophysiological mechanisms of SSNHL. Such a complex disease is to consider a multifactorial and polygenic condition in which gene-environment interactions have a key role. In particular, considering the possible link between iron metabolism and inner ear oxidative stress, more efforts should be performed in order to better understand the complex biochemical environment and mechanisms of the inner ear.

References

[1] Nakashima T, Itoh A, Misawa H, Ohno Y. Clinicoepidemiologic features of sudden deafness diagnosed and treated at university hospitals in Japan. *Otolaryngol Head Neck Surg.* 2000;123(5):593-7.

[2] Olzowy B, Osterkorn D, Suckfull M. [The incidence of sudden hearing loss is greater than previously assumed]. *MMW Fortschritte der Medizin.* 2005;147(14):37-8.

[3] Aimoni C, Bianchini C, Borin M, Ciorba A, Fellin R, Martini A, et al. Diabetes, cardiovascular risk factors and idiopathic sudden sensorineural hearing loss: a case-control study. *Audiol Neurootol.* 2010;15(2):111-5.

[4] Zajtchuk JT, Falor WH, Jr., Rhodes MF. Hypercoagulability as a cause of sudden neurosensory hearing loss. *Otolaryngology and head and neck surgery.* 1979;87(2):268-73.

[5] Yildiz Z, Ulu A, Incesulu A, Ozkaptan Y, Akar N. The importance of thrombotic risk factors in the development of idiopathic sudden hearing loss. *Clinical and applied thrombosis/hemostasis: Official journal of the International Academy of Clinical and Applied Thrombosis/Hemostasis.* 2008;14(3):356-9.

[6] Yoon TH, Paparella MM, Schachern PA, Alleva M. Histopathology of sudden hearing loss. *The Laryngoscope.* 1990;100(7):707-15.

[7] Garrick MD. Human iron transporters. *Genes & nutrition.* 2011;6(1):45-54.

[8] Zheng G, Chen J, Zheng W. Relative contribution of CTR1 and DMT1 in copper transport by the blood-CSF barrier: implication in manganese-induced neurotoxicity. *Toxicology and applied pharmacology.* 2012;260(3):285-93.

[9] Liu X, Zheng G, Wu Y, Shen X, Jing J, Yu T, et al. Lead exposure results in hearing loss and disruption of the cochlear blood-labyrinth barrier and the protective role of iron supplement. *Neurotoxicology.* 2013;39:173-81.

[10] Gemmati D, Zeri G, Orioli E, De Gaetano FE, Salvi F, Bartolomei I, et al. Polymorphisms in the genes coding for iron binding and transporting proteins are associated with disability, severity, and early progression in multiple sclerosis. *BMC medical genetics.* 2012;13:70.

[11] Williams BB, Kwakye GF, Wegrzynowicz M, Li D, Aschner M, Erikson KM, et al. Altered manganese homeostasis and manganese toxicity in a Huntington's disease striatal cell model are not explained by defects in the iron transport system. *Toxicological sciences : an official journal of the Society of Toxicology.* 2010;117(1):169-79.

[12] Mills E, Dong XP, Wang F, Xu H. Mechanisms of brain iron transport: insight into neurodegeneration and CNS disorders. *Future medicinal chemistry.* 2010;2(1):51-64.

[13] Gemmati D, Federici F, Catozzi L, Gianesini S, Tacconi G, Scapoli GL, et al. DNA-array of gene variants in venous leg ulcers: detection of prognostic indicators. *Journal of vascular surgery.* 2009;50(6):1444-51.

[14] Zamboni P, Izzo M, Tognazzo S, Carandina S, De Palma M, Catozzi L, et al. The overlapping of local iron overload and HFE mutation in venous leg ulcer pathogenesis. *Free radical biology & medicine.* 2006;40(10):1869-73.

[15] Yamasoba T, Sakai K, Sakurai M. Role of acute cochlear neuritis in sudden hearing loss in multiple sclerosis. *Journal of the neurological sciences.* 1997;146(2):179-81.

[16] Wink DA, Hines HB, Cheng RY, Switzer CH, Flores-Santana W, Vitek MP, et al. Nitric oxide and redox mechanisms in the immune response. *Journal of leukocyte biology.* 2011;89(6):873-91.

[17] Brissot P, Ropert M, Le Lan C, Loreal O. Non-transferrin bound iron: a key role in iron overload and iron toxicity. Biochimica *et biophysica acta.* 2012;1820(3):403-10.

[18] Singh R, Wangemann P. Free radical stress-mediated loss of Kcnj10 protein expression in stria vascularis contributes to deafness in Pendred syndrome mouse model. *American journal of physiology Renal physiology.* 2008;294(1):F139-48.

[19] Singh AV, Subhashree L, Milani P, Gemmati D, Zamboni P. Interplay of iron metallobiology, metalloproteinases, and FXIII, and role of their gene variants in venous leg ulcer. *The international journal of lower extremity wounds.* 2010;9(4):166-79.

[20] Sun AH, Wang ZM, Xiao SZ, Li ZJ, Ding JC, Li JY, et al. Idiopathic sudden hearing loss and disturbance of iron metabolism. A clinical survey of 426 cases. ORL; *Journal for oto-rhino-laryngology and its related specialties.* 1992;54(2):66-70.

[21] Sun AH, Wang ZM, Xiao SZ, Li ZJ, Zheng Z, Li JY. Sudden sensorineural hearing loss induced by experimental iron deficiency in rats. ORL; *Journal for oto-rhino-laryngology and its related specialties.* 1992;54(5):246-50.

[22] Hanninen MM, Haapasalo J, Haapasalo H, Fleming RE, Britton RS, Bacon BR, et al. Expression of iron-related genes in human brain and brain tumors. *BMC neuroscience.* 2009;10:36.

[23] Johnstone D, Graham RM, Trinder D, Delima RD, Riveros C, Olynyk JK, et al. Brain transcriptome perturbations in the Hfe(-/-) mouse model of genetic iron loading. *Brain research.* 2012;1448:144-52.

[24] Mao J, McKean DM, Warrier S, Corbin JG, Niswander L, Zohn IE. The iron exporter ferroportin 1 is essential for development of the mouse embryo, forebrain patterning and neural tube closure. *Development.* 2010;137(18):3079-88.

[25] Bai SP, Lu L, Luo XG, Liu B. Cloning, sequencing, characterization, and expressions of divalent metal transporter one in the small intestine of broilers. *Poultry science.* 2008;87(4):768-76.
[26] Ward DM, Kaplan J. Ferroportin-mediated iron transport: expression and regulation. *Biochimica et biophysica acta.* 2012;1823(9):1426-33.
[27] Gardenghi S, Marongiu MF, Ramos P, Guy E, Breda L, Chadburn A, et al. Ineffective erythropoiesis in beta-thalassemia is characterized by increased iron absorption mediated by down-regulation of hepcidin and up regulation of ferroportin. *Blood.* 2007;109(11):5027-35.
[28] Troadec MB, Ward DM, Lo E, Kaplan J, De Domenico I. Induction of FPN1 transcription by MTF-1 reveals a role for ferroportin in transition metal efflux. *Blood.* 2010;116(22):4657-64.
[29] Zhang DL, Senecal T, Ghosh MC, Ollivierre-Wilson H, Tu T, Rouault TA. Hepcidin regulates ferroportin expression and intracellular iron homeostasis of erythroblasts. *Blood.* 2011;118(10):2868-77.
[30] Ganz T. Molecular control of iron transport. Journal of the American Society of Nephrology : *JASN.* 2007;18(2):394-400.
[31] Ding H, Yan CZ, Shi H, Zhao YS, Chang SY, Yu P, et al. Hepcidin is involved in iron regulation in the ischemic brain. *PloS one.* 2011;6(9):e25324.
[32] Haberkamp TJ, Tanyeri HM. Management of idiopathic sudden sensorineural hearing loss. *Am J Otol.* 1999;20(5):587-92; discussion 93-5.
[33] Clark JG. Uses and abuses of hearing loss classification. *Asha.* 1981;23(7):493-500.
[34] Tran Ba Huy P, Sauvaget E. [Idiopathic sudden sensorineural hearing loss is not, at this time, an otologic emergency]. *Ann Otolaryngol Chir Cervicofac.* 2007;124(2):66-71.
[35] Young YH, Lou PJ. Post-irradiation sudden deafness. *J Laryngol Otol.* 1999;113(9):815-7.
[36] Yossepowitch O, Lossos A, Lossos IS. Sudden hearing loss following acute hepatitis. *Postgraduate medical journal.* 1999;75(883):309-12.
[37] Yoshimoto Y. Clinico-statistical study on acoustic tumors with sudden hearing loss. *Auris Nasus Larynx.* 1988;15(3):165-71.
[38] Yin T, Huang F, Ren J, Liu W, Chen X, Li L, et al. Bilateral sudden hearing loss following habitual abortion: a case report and review of literature. *International journal of clinical and experimental medicine.* 2013;6(8):720-3.
[39] Uchida Y, Sugiura S, Ando F, Shimokata H, Nakashima T. Association of the C677T polymorphism in the methylenetetrahydrofolate reductase gene with sudden sensorineural hearing loss. *The Laryngoscope.* 2010;120(4):791-5.
[40] Uchida Y, Sugiura S, Nakashima T, Ando F, Shimokata H. Contribution of 1425G/A polymorphism in protein kinase C-Eta (PRKCH) gene and brain white matter lesions to the risk of sudden sensorineural hearing loss in a Japanese nested case-control study. *Journal of neurogenetics.* 2011;25(3):82-7.
[41] Uchida Y, Teranishi M, Nishio N, Sugiura S, Hiramatsu M, Suzuki H, et al. Endothelin-1 gene polymorphism in sudden sensorineural hearing loss. *The Laryngoscope.* 2013;123(11):E59-65.
[42] Teranishi M, Uchida Y, Nishio N, Kato K, Otake H, Yoshida T, et al. Polymorphisms in genes involved in the free-radical process in patients with sudden sensorineural hearing loss and Meniere's disease. *Free radical research.* 2013;47(6-7):498-506.

[43] Capaccio P, Ottaviani F, Cuccarini V, Ambrosetti U, Fagnani E, Bottero A, et al. Sudden hearing loss and MTHFR 677C>T/1298A>C gene polymorphisms. Genetics in medicine : *official journal of the American College of Medical Genetics.* 2005;7(3):206-8.

[44] Cho SH, Chen H, Kim IS, Yokose C, Kang J, Cho D, et al. Association of the 4 g/5 g polymorphism of plasminogen activator inhibitor-1 gene with sudden sensorineural hearing loss. A case control study. *BMC ear, nose, and throat disorders.* 2012;12:5.

[45] Zhang Z, Zhang F, An P, Guo X, Shen Y, Tao Y, et al. Ferroportin1 deficiency in mouse macrophages impairs iron homeostasis and inflammatory responses. *Blood.* 2011;118(7):1912-22.

[46] Liu X-b, Hill P, Haile DJ. Role of the Ferroportin Iron-Responsive Element in Iron and Nitric Oxide Dependent Gene Regulation. Blood Cells, *Molecules, and Diseases.* 2002;29(3):315-26.

[47] Santos-Sacchi J, Marovitz WF. A ferritin-containing cell type in the stria vascularis of the mouse inner ear. *Acta Otolaryngol.* 1985;100(1-2):26-32.

[48] Ding D, Salvi R, Roth JA. Cellular localization and developmental changes of the different isoforms of divalent metal transporter 1 (DMT1) in the inner ear of rats. *Biometals : an international journal on the role of metal ions in biology, biochemistry, and medicine.* 2013.

[49] Mazurek B, Amarjargal N, Haupt H, Fuchs J, Olze H, Machulik A, et al. Expression of genes implicated in oxidative stress in the cochlea of newborn rats. *Hearing research.* 2011;277(1-2):54-60.

[50] Marcus DC, Thalmann R, Marcus NY. Respiratory rate and ATP content of stria vascularis of guinea pig in vitro. *The Laryngoscope.* 1978;88(11):1825-35.

[51] Hansen JB, Tonnesen MF, Madsen AN, Hagedorn PH, Friberg J, Grunnet LG, et al. Divalent metal transporter 1 regulates iron-mediated ROS and pancreatic beta cell fate in response to cytokines. *Cell metabolism.* 2012;16(4):449-61.

[52] Abouhamed M, Wolff NA, Lee WK, Smith CP, Thevenod F. Knockdown of endosomal/lysosomal divalent metal transporter 1 by RNA interference prevents cadmium-metallothionein-1 cytotoxicity in renal proximal tubule cells. American journal of physiology *Renal physiology.* 2007;293(3):F705-12.

[53] Chung SD, Chen PY, Lin HC, Hung SH. Sudden sensorineural hearing loss associated with iron-deficiency anemia: a population-based study. *JAMA Otolaryngol Head Neck Surg.* 2014 May;140(5):417-22.

[54] Sun AH,Wang ZM, Xiao SZ, et al. Idiopathic sudden hearing loss and disturbance of iron metabolism: a clinical survey of 426 cases. *ORL J Otorhinolaryngol Relat Spec.* 1992;54(2):66-70.

In: Handbook of Hearing Disorders Research
Editor: Charlotte Hailee Atkinson
ISBN: 978-1-63463-654-4

Chapter 4

Association between Sensorineural Hearing Loss and Sleep-disordered Breathing: Literature Review

Antonella Ballacchino[1], Rosalia Gargano[2] and Francesco Martines[2]

[1]Università degli Studi di Palermo, Dipartimento di Biotecnologie Mediche e Medicina Forenze Sezione di Audiologia, Palermo, Italy

[2]Università degli Studi di Palermo, Dipartimento di Biomedicina Sperimentale e Neuroscienze Cliniche, Sezione di Otorinolaringoiatria, Palermo, Italy

Abstract

The cochlea is especially sensitive to circulatory alterations because it is supplied by a single terminal artery and lacks adequate collateral blood supply.

To examine the putative association between Sensorineural Hearing Loss (SNHL) and Sleep Disordered Breathing (SDB) through the literature review is very interesting.

In fact these medical disorders usually are associated to cerebral circulatory alterations resulting in hypoxia, acute hemodynamic change, and decreased cerebral blood flow, because the Sleep Disorder Breathing (SDB), for example OSAHS (Obstructive Sleep Apnea Hypopnea Syndrome), is characterized by periodic hyposia/reoxygenation. These noxious stimuli can, in turn, activate the sympathetic nervous system, depress parasympathetic activity which results in oxidative stress, endothelial dysfunction, and activation of the inflammatory cascade of different anatomical structure as inner ear. Is reasonable to assume that could cause and/or esacerbate sensorineural hearing loss with/or without tinnitus.

Based on these clinical evidences some authors studied the association between SDB and a dysfunction of auditory pathway showing an improved risk of sensorineural hearing loss, a lower transient otoacoustic emissions (TEOAE) reproducibility and an impairment of auditory brainstem responses in OSAHS populatio. In fact it is known that the transduction mechanism of the inner ear and the transmission of nerve impulses along the auditory way are highly dependent upon the oxygen supply. Recent studies evidenced how through oxidative injury due to a hypoxic stress induced apoptosis in spiral ligament and in the cochlear basal turn of the Organ of Corti of obese CD/1 mouses, causes a high frequencies sensorineural hearing loss.

Therefore OSAHS may lead to cerebral vascular insufficiency resulting in hypoxia, acute hemodynamic change, and decreased cerebral blood flow during episodes of apnea with consequent ischemic injury to the cochlea.

Keywords: Sensorineural Hearing Loss (SNHL), Sleep Disordered Breathing (SDB), Hypoxia, OSAHS (Obstructive Sleep Apnea Hypopnea Syndrome), Endothelial dysfunction

Introduction

Sleep Disordered breathing (SDB), including Obstructive Sleep Apnea Hypopnea Syndrome (OSAHS) is a condition, affecting 24% of men and 9% of women in their middle age, associated to high values either of Body Mass Index (BMI) and neck circumference, where intermittent obstruction of the airway during sleep causes sleep fragmentation and repeated desaturations. This disorder carries potentially serious consequences: excessive daytime sleepiness, neurocognitive deterioration, endocrine and metabolic derangements, and is universally recognized as independent risk factor for cardiovascular disease and its related mortality [1-3]. Ear hypoxia is linked to damage of cochlear structures, vascular streaks, afferent synapses, internal ciliated cells but above all it is external ciliated cells of the basal turn which seem most vulnerable: this damage is responsible for sensorineural hearing loss and tinnitus [4-9]. These phenomena lead to a chronic state of oxidative stress resulting in endothelial inflammation, in fact some studies estimated that in patients with sleep-related breathing disorders the probability of a cerebral vascular infarction (CVI) is 3.1 times that in patients without sleep apnea and that 25-50% of all patients who have a stroke suffer from sleep apnea (OSAHS) and have a respiratory disturbance index (RDI) higher than 10. CVI may be caused by variations in intracranial pressure or in intracranial hemodynamics owing to decreasing pO(2) and increasing pCO(2) during cessation of airflow. It is suspected that the most common causes of sudden deafness are vasospasm, thrombosis, embolism, hypercoagulation and sludging [10-15].

Basing on these clinical evidences some authors studied the association between OSAHS and a dysfunction of auditory pathway showing an improved risk of sudden sensorineural hearing loss (SSNHL), a lower transient otoacoustic emissions (TEOAE) reproducibility and an impairment of auditory brainstem responses in OSAHS population [16,17].

What Are the Mechanisms that Determine the Audiological Damage in Patients with SDB?

The transduction mechanism of the inner ear and the transmission of nerve impulses along the auditory way are highly dependent upon the cochlear oxygen supply,

SDB, in particular OSAHS, is characterised by repetitive airway occlusion resulting in cyclical surges of hypoxia which may occur hundreds of times a night. In addition, OSAHS is associated with heart failure, stroke and coronary artery disease [18-22]. Endothelial dysfunction, linked to oxidative stress ("Oxidative stress" is the general phenomenon of oxidant exposure and antioxidant depletion, or oxidant-antioxidant balance), a key early event in hypertension and atherosclerosis, has been implicated as a possible mechanism linking the acute cyclical vascular stresses during sleep in OSAHS and the increased prevalence of chronic vascular diseases. Oxidative stress may induce neurotoxicity phenomena that lead to neurodegeneration. As the hair cells of Corti is particularly sensitive to oxidative stress, especially at the mitochondrial level, can go more easily meet degeneration or cell death (disorganization of cochlear homeostasis induced), resulting in an irreversible hearing damage [23]. In addition, the metabolic implications in common with hearing disorders and SDB are obvious, in fact, one of the most important is that anoxia during OSAHS is a potent stimulus for catecholamine secretion and glycogenolysis. An indirect effect regards obesity, as it is tightly connected with diabetes (to emphasize this connection the term "diabesity" has been created) [24,25]. There are also some studies that demonstrate the increase of inflammatory factors in subjects with OSASH: among these, C-reactive protein and cytokines, which are responsible for systemic atherosclerosis and probably have a role in the appearance of neoplasms [26,27] and also evidence of an increase of atherogenic dyslipidaemia [28,29]. Hyperlipidemia determines, at the level of small vessels, a suffering of flow related to increased blood viscosity. This results in a reduced supply of oxygen to the inner ear and its suffering.

Literature Review

Many authors investigated the epidemiologic association between OSAHS and either sudden SNHL and dysfunction of auditory pathway. In a study of Fischer et al. a 7-channel polygraph was used to test 33 subjects with normal hearing and 27 patients suffering from sudden hearing loss and found that 29.6% of the patient group and 21.2% of those in the study control group were suffering from OSA and had RDI >10; this difference was not significant (p=0.554). Sudden hearing loss may also be an indicator of arteriosclerosis secondary to such risk factors as hypertension (p=0.005), diabetes (p=0.003), and hyperlipidemia (p=0.004), which were highly significant for the patient group [10]. Sheu et al. evidenced how in a case-control study performed on 19152 patients, OSAHS is present on 1.7% of SSNHL population respect to the 1.2% of the controls with a significant difference between the groups (P<0.04) [16]. Recently Casale et al. studied 30 patients divided in two groups, cases (18 subjects) with severe OSA and controls (21 subjects) with snoring without OSAHS and evidenced higher mean values at pure tone audiogram and lower TEOAE signal to noise ratio in severe OSAHS group with significant differences among cases and controls (P<0.01) [17]. The authors suggested as possible explanation for the association between SDB and SSNHL, that OSAHS indirectly contributes to the development of SSNHL, the effects of cardiovascular disease and cardiovascular risk factors and that is associated with reduced basal and functional capillarity rarefaction with an additional risk of impaired peripheral perfusion and therefore dysfunction of cochlear hair cells [16,17].

Hwang et al. evidenced how through oxidative injury due to a hypoxic stress induced apoptosis in spiral ligament and in the cochlear basal turn of the Organ of Corti of obese CD/1 mouses, causes a high frequencies sensorineural hearing loss [30]; as also demonstrated by a study of CAO Yongmao et al. which analyzed the hearing at extended high frequencies of patients with obstructive sleep apnea-hyponea syndrome. The youth group, adult group and OSAHS group were tested with pure tone audiometry and high frequency audiometry, and the res ponse ratio was calculated [31]. The conclusion was: the high frequency thresholds increased obviously when OSAHS group comparing with the adult group (P0.01), and the indicating ratio decreased obviously (P 0.05) [31].

One of the most interesting studies on this topic was conducted by Jau-Jiuan Sheu et al., in this case-control study, identified 3192 patients diagnosed with SSNHL from the Taiwan Longitudinal Health Insurance Database as the study group and randomly extracted the data of 15 960 subjects matched by sex, age and year of first SSNHL diagnosis as controls. Of 19 152 patients, 1.2% had OSA diagnoses prior to the index date; OSA was diagnosed in 1.7% of the SSNHL group and 1.2% of the controls. After adjusting for sociodemographic characteristics and comorbid medical disorders, we found that male patients with SSNHL were more likely to have prior OSA than controls (odds ratio, 1.48; 95% CI, 1.02-2.16) (*P*=.04) [32]. Dziewas et al. in a study performed in 2007 showed how the recurrent intermittent hypoxaemia may be considered a risk factor for peripheral sensory nerve dysfunction and suggested that the treatment for OSAHS might result in an improved function of these nerves [33].

Conclusion

The cochlea is especially sensitive to circulatory alterations because it is supplied by a single terminal artery and lacks adequate collateral blood supply [34]. Obstructive sleep apnea may lead to cerebral vascular insufficiency resulting in hypoxia, acute hemodynamic change, and decreased cerebral blood flow during episodes of apnea [2]. In addition, elevated sympathetic nerve activity secondary to the reflex effects of hypoxia and hypercapnia as well as oscillations in blood pressure occurring during episodes of apnea may result in adverse cerebrovascular events and hence ischemic injury to the cochlea [35].

The correlations between SDB and hearing disorders are widely demonstrated in the literature and is still studied.

The presence of sensorineural hearing loss associated with essential hypertension, high cholesterol and high BMI should suspect the presence of SDB misunderstood. This would allow an early diagnosis of these disorders, the resolution of hearing loss and protection to cardiovascular and cerebrovascular accidents.

In fact the early treatment of OSAHS with CPAP (continuous positive airway pressure) improves systemic vascular endothelial function. OSAHS has been implicated in the pathogenesis of hypertension, cardiovascular disease, heart failure, and stroke, all of which are associated with impaired endothelial responses. CPAP treatment may therefore provide an opportunity to reduce the vascular risk attributable to OSAHS, as well as hearing loss, allowing a better and continuous oxygenation of the blood vessels smaller [36].

References

[1] Bradley TD, Floras JS (2009). Obstructive sleep apnoea and its cardiovascular consequences. *Lancet* 373:82–93 286.

[2] Redline S, Tishler P (2003). The genetics of sleep apnea. *Sleep Med Rev* 4:583–602.

[3] Fletcher EC (1995). The relationship between systemic hypertension and obstructive sleep apnea: facts and theory. *Am J Med* 98:118–128.

[4] Morris L, Kleinberger A, Lee K, et al. (2008). Rapid risk stratification for obstructive sleep apnea, based on snoring severity and body mass index. *Otolaryngology-Head and Neck Surgery*; 139: 615-618.

[5] Rebillard G, Lavigne-Rebillard M. Effect of reversible hypoxia on the compared time courses of endocochlear potential and 2f1-f2 distortion products, (1992) *Hearing Reserch*; 62(2) : 142-148.

[6] Martines F, Sireci F, Cannizzaro E et al, (2014). Clinical observations and risk factors for tinnitus in a Sicilian cohort. *Eur Arch Otorhinolaryngol.*; Sep. 5; DOI 10.1007/s00405-014-3275-0.

[7] Salvago P, Martines E, Martines F, (2013). Prevalence and risk factors for sensorineural hearing loss: Western Sicily overview. *Eur Arch Otorhinolaryngol.*; 270:3049–56.

[8] Martines F, Bentivegna D, Martines E et al, (2010). Assessing audiological, pathophysiological and psychological variables in tinnitus patients with or without hearing loss. *Eur Arch Otorhinolaryngol.*; 267:1685-1693

[9] Martines F, Bentivegna D, Martines E et al, (2010). Characteristics of tinnitus with or without hearing loss: clinical observations in Sicilian tinnitus patients. *Auris Nasus Larynx*; 37:685-693.

[10] Fischer Y, Yakinthou A, (2003 Jun). Prevalence of obstructive sleep apnea syndrome (OSA) in patients with sudden hearing loss. A pilot study. *WJ. HNO.*; 51(6):462-6.

[11] Martines F, Maira E, Ferrara S, (2011). Age related hearing impairment (ARHI): a common sensory deficit in the elderly. *Acta Medica Mediterranea*; 27:47–52.

[12] Martines F, Dispenza F, Gagliardo C, Martines E, Bentivegna D, (2011). Sudden sensorineural hearing loss as prodromal symptom of anterior inferior cerebellar artery infarction. *ORL*; 73:137–40.

[13] Martines F, Martinciglio G, Bucalo C et al, (2008). Neurovascular conflict in patient with tinnitus and essential hypertension: case report. *Otorinolaringol*; 58: *191-196.*

[14] Gagliardo C, Martines F, Bencivinni F, (2013). Intratumoral Haemorrhage Causing an Unusual Clinical Presentation of a Vestibular Schwannoma. *Neuroradiol J.;* 26(1):30-4.

[15] Martines F, Agrifoglio M, Bentivegna D, (2012). Treatment of tinnitus and dizziness associated vertebrobasilar insufficiency with a fixed combination of cinnarizine and dimenhydrinate. *Acta Medica Mediterranea*; 28:291–296.

[16] Sheu JJ, Wu CS, Lin HC, (2012). Association Between Obstructive Sleep Apnea and Sudden Sensorineural Hearing Loss. A Population-Based Case-Control Study. *Arch Otolaryngol Head Neck Surg.*;138(1):55-9.

[17] Casale M, Vesperini E, Potena M, Pappacena M, Bressi F, Baptista PJ, Salvinelli F, (2012). Is obstructive sleep apnea syndrome a risk factor for auditory pathway? *Sleep Breath* 16:413–417.

[18] Javaheri S, Parker TJ, Liming JD, et al. (1998). Sleep apnea in 81 ambulatory malepatients with stable heart failure. Types and their prevalences, consequences, and presentations. *Circulation*; 97:2154–2159.

[19] Dyken ME, Somers VK, Yamada T, e al. (1996). Investigating the relationship between stroke and obstructive sleep apnea. *Stroke*; 27:401–407.

[20] Wessendorf TE, Teschler H, Wang YM, et al. (2000) Sleep-disordered breathing among patients with first-ever stroke. *J Neurol;* 247:41–47.

[21] Hung J, Whitford EG, Parsons RW, et al. (1990). Association of sleep apnoea with myocardial infarction in men. *Lancet*; 336:261–264.

[22] Peker Y, Kraiczi H, Hedner J, et al. (1999). An independent association between obstructive sleep apnoea and coronary artery disease. *Eur Respir J*;14:179–84.

[23] Serra A, Maiolino L, (2011). Ruolo delle Biossidazione nelle patologie dell'orecchio interno. *Argomenti di acta otorhinolaryngologica italica*, vol. 5, no2, pp. 7-9.

[24] Tatti B, Passali D, Bellussi L.M, (2012). The undisclosed role of anoxia/hypoxia and disturbed sleep on glucose metabolism. *J Diabete Mellitus*; 2:186-90.

[25] Spiegel K, (2004). Sleep curtailment in healthy young men is associated with decreased leptin levels, elevated ghrelin levels, and increased hunger and appetite; *Ann Internal Med*;141:846-50.

[26] Passali D, Tatti P, Passali F.M, et al. (2013). The undisclosed role of disturbed sleep and hypoxia on metabolism: the importance of upper airways pathology. *Sleep Breath*;17:5-6.

[27] Popko K, Gorska E, Potapinska O, et al. (2008). Frequency of dis- tribution of inflammatory cytokines IL-1, IL-6 and TNF-gene polymorphism in patients with obstructive sleep apnea. *J Physiol Pharmacol*; 59 (Suppl. 6):607-14.

[28] Ciftci TU, Kokturk O, Bukan N, et al. (2004) The relationship between serum cytokine levels with obesity and obstructive sleep apnea syndrome. *Cytokine*; 28:87-91.

[29] Williams CJ, Hu FB, Patel SR, et al. (2007). Sleep duration and snoring in relation to cardiovascular disease risk in women with type 2 diabetes. *Diabetes Care*; 30:1233-40.

[30] Hwang JH, Hsu CJ, Yu TC, et al. (2013). Diet-Induced Obesity Exacerbates Auditory Degeneration via Hypoxia, Inflammation, and Apoptosis Signaling Pathways in CD/1 Mice. *PLoS ONE*, vol. 8, issue 4, p. e60730.

[31] Cao Y, Luo Z, Tao Z, et al. (2006). Analysis of the hearing of patients with obstructive sleep apnea-hypopnea syndrome. *Journal of Clinical Otorhinolaryngology Head and Neck Surgery* 1001-1781 Issue 1.

[32] Sheu JJ, Wu CS, Lin HC, (2012). Association Between Obstructive Sleep Apnea and Sudden Sensorineural Hearing Loss. A Population-Based Case-Control Study. *Arch Otolaryngol Head Neck Surg.*; 138(1):55-59.

[33] Dziewas R, Schilling M, Engel P, Boentert M, Hor H, Okegwo A, Lüdemann P, Ringelstein EB, Young P (2007) Treatment for obstructive sleep apnoea: effect on peripheral nerve function. *J Neurol Neurosurg Psychiatr* 78:295–297

[34] Gross JB, Bachenberg KL, Benumof JL, (2006). Practice guidelines for the perioperative management of patients with obstructive sleep apnea: a report by the American Society of Anesthesiologists Task Force on Perioperative Management of patients with obstructive sleep apnea. *Anesthesiology*;104:1081-93.

[35] Chung F, Subramanyam R, Liao P, et al, (2012). High STOP-Bang score indicates a high probability of obstructive sleep apnoea. *Br J Anaesth*: 108(5):768-775.

[36] Lattimore JL, Wilcox I, Skilton M, et al. (2006). Treatment of obstructive sleep apnoea leads to improved microvascular endothelial function in the systemic circulation. *Thorax*; 61:491–495.

In: Handbook of Hearing Disorders Research
Editor: Charlotte Hailee Atkinson
ISBN: 978-1-63463-654-4

Chapter 5

Chronic Tinnitus: Pith, Loudness, and Discomfort in Adults and Elderly Patients

Adriane Ribeiro Teixeira[1],*
Letícia Petersen Schmidt Rosito,[2]
Bruna Macagnin Seimetz,[3] *Celso Dall'Igna*[4]
and Sady Selaimen da Costa [5]

[1]Audiologist, Doctorade in Biomedical Gerontology, Professor in Department of Human and Communication Disorders, Federal University of Rio Grande do Sul, Brazil
[2]Medical Otorhinolaryngologist, Doctorate in Medicine: Surgical Clinic, Hospital Clinics of Porto Alegre, Brazil
[3]Speech therapist and Audiologist, Master's Degree in Health of Children and Adolescents, Federal University of Rio Grande do Sul, Brazil
[4]Medical Otorhinolaryngologist, Doctorate in Respiratory Sciences, Professor in Department of Ophthalmology and Otorhinolaryngology – Federal University of Rio Grande do Sul, Brazil
[5]Medical Otorhinolaryngologist, Doctorate in Medicine: Surgical Clinic, Professor in Department of Ophthalmology and Otorhinolaryngology, Federal University of Rio Grande do Sul, Brazil

Abstract

Tinnitus is a common symptom in individuals of various age groups, but the impact it causes is variable, depending on the characteristics of subjects. The aim of this study is to analyze the characteristics of tinnitus and the discomfort it causes in individuals assessed in a specific outpatient clinic in a tertiary hospital. Participants were evaluated

* Corresponding author's email: adriane.teixeira@gmail.com.

by medical history interview, medical examination, grading of tinnitus severity, hearing screening and testing, measurement of tinnitus pitch and loudness and THI instrument for identifying tinnitus discomfort. The sample consisted of 199 individuals; 124 of them (62.30%) were females, with a mean age of 58.18 ± 12.79 years, with bilateral tinnitus (50.8%) and average length of tinnitus presence was 5.18 ± 4.67 years. Tinnitus pitch was acute and tinnitus loudness was moderate, within the values reported in the technical literature. Mean tinnitus severity was 5.18 ± 4.67 years and the THI score ranged from 0 to 98 points (mean 40.03 ± 25.48 points). No difference was observed between THI scores and sex and tinnitus location. Correlation was observed between tinnitus severity and THI scores, between age and tinnitus loudness in the left ear, and between age and THI scores.

Introduction

Tinnitus is a common symptom in medical and audiological exams. It is defined as the sound perceived by the subject without an external source being present. [1, 2] It may be caused by otological, neurological, cardiovascular, rheumatological, endocrine, metabolic and immune diseases. Trauma, temporomandibular joint disorders, psychological problems and use of ototoxic medication are also causes of tinnitus. [2, 3]

Tinnitus can be graded in several ways. Tinnitus can be considered as subjective (perceived only by the affected individual) or objective (perceived by others), continuous or intermittent, pulsatile or non-pulsatile, unilateral or bilateral or located in the center of the head. The onset may be sudden or insidious. [2, 4] Grading is used by health professionals to categorize the symptom as shown by individuals. It assists in determining etiology and treatment.

The prevalence of tinnitus varies depending on the population studied. A study conducted in South Korea showed that 19.7% of individuals aged 12 years or older had the symptom. [5] Another study with Japanese elderly showed that 18.7% of them had tinnitus. [6] In Egypt, the prevalence was 5.17% and in the United States, 25.3%. [7, 8] The prevalence of tinnitus in the elderly is higher than in adults, with values ranging between 33% and 72.5%. [9,10] General data show that in 2004, tinnitus affected 15% of the world population, [11] and its prevalence increased to 25.3% in 2012. [12]

Although it is a more frequent complaint by adults and the elderly, children can also have tinnitus. Research conducted in Brazil showed a high prevalence of tinnitus in children. In a study that evaluated 477 children, continuous tinnitus was found in 21.7% and pulsatile tinnitus in 3.8% of them. [13] Another more recent study showed that 54.7% of the children interviewed had had tinnitus for the past 12 months. [12]

The relationship between tinnitus and gender of affected individuals is still controversial in the literature. [14] Some studies showed a similar number of affected individuals, [6, 14] while others showed a higher prevalence of women [10, 15, 16] or men. [17, 18, 19]

Despite the high prevalence of tinnitus, the discomfort it causes is variable, because some individuals reported tinnitus but their activities were not affected by the symptom, while others reported severe problems. [2, 19] It is believed that approximately 20% of tinnitus patients feel discomfort. [20] Factors such as personality traits, depression, anxiety, difficulty in dealing with problems, and concentration difficulties influence the level of discomfort caused by tinnitus. [21, 22] It is actually a prognostic factor for treatment.[23] Thus, primary psychological factors influence the level of discomfort and the result in the treatment of tinnitus. [4, 14, 20] Patients' concern about tinnitus is crucial for adapting to it, and there may be a vicious circle that patients cannot cope with. [14]

On the same line of reasoning, depression can be caused by tinnitus, but it can also be indicative of poor adaptation to it. [24] Likewise, sleep disorders may be caused by tinnitus, but they could also exist prior to the appearance of the symptom, i.e. they could be a comorbidity rather than a consequence of it. [14] These and other disorders (anxiety and stress, for example) lead to loss of quality of life, which is widely described in the literature. [2, 23, 25, 26] However, in a study with subjects outside the hospital or clinical environment, there was no influence of tinnitus on quality of life. [17] This seems to reinforce the idea that the discomfort and the consequences of tinnitus are related to the psychological aspects of individuals.

Research conducted to date showed no influence of the variables age and gender on discomfort caused by tinnitus. [14, 20]

The evaluation of individuals with tinnitus aims to define the etiology and treatment of it. It is supposed to include detailed history, physical examination, laboratory tests, audiological evaluation and radiological assessment. [27] Moreover, questionnaires should be used to determine the impact of tinnitus on a patient's life. The Tinnitus Handicap Inventory (THI) is one of the most used, and it has already been translated, adapted and validated into several languages. Originally created in the English language, [28] it has versions in Brazilian Portuguese [29], Chinese - Mandarin and Cantonese [30, 31], French, [32] Italian, [33] Spanish, [34] Filipino [35] and Persian, [36] among others.

THI is composed of 25 questions for assessing the effects of tinnitus in the restriction of daily activities of affected individuals. [37] There are three types of response for each situation: Yes (4 points), Sometimes (2 points) or No (0 points). The sum of points obtained in each response allows one to assess the level of discomfort caused by the symptom: slight (0-16 points), mild (18-36 points), moderate (38-56 points), severe (58 to 76 points) and catastrophic (78-100 points). [14] Because it is quick and easy to apply and interpret, addresses the influence of tinnitus on a patient's life, and has adequate validity and reliability, THI is routinely used in the clinical evaluation of patients. [28, 38]

Although tinnitus is studied by researchers from various countries, further research about tinnitus and its effects is still needed, especially in light of the contradictions in the literature. Thus, the objective of this study is to analyze the characteristics of tinnitus and the discomfort it causes in subjects evaluated in a specific outpatient clinic in a tertiary hospital.

Methodology

This was a cross-sectional study conducted in a tertiary care hospital in southern Brazil. The sample consisted of both male and female patients suffering from chronic tinnitus and history of tinnitus discomfort, who were seen in a specific outpatient clinic. The presence of the symptom for a period of time greater than six months was defined as chronic tinnitus. [26]

Patients were evaluated by otolaryngologists and audiologists who determine the presence of hearing loss, tinnitus characteristics, the etiology of it and the presence of other comorbidities, such as depression, anxiety, metabolic disorders, etc.

ENT evaluation consisted of medical history interview, physical examination and otoscopy. After that, patients wree evaluated by audiologists through pure tone audiometry testing of hearing thresholds for high frequencies and conventional frequencies, speech audiometry, acuphenometry, measurement of loudness discomfort levels and acoustic immitance. Next, patients underwent laboratory tests and imaging tests, if necessary.

The medical history interview, conducted through oral questions to be answered by patients, investigated sociodemographic data (age, gender, race), health history (diseases, medication use) and tinnitus history (length of symptom presence, laterality, improvement or worsening factors, etc.). Patients were also asked about tinnitus severity. Patients were asked: "On a 0-10 scale, how much does tinnitus bother you in your life?". After that, the version of the THI instrument that was validated and translated into Portuguese. [29]

Then, patients underwent audiological evaluation, and a complete audiological evaluation was made. At first, all patients underwent pure tone audiometry; conventional frequencies and high frequencies were measured. The examination was conducted in a soundproof booth, and thresholds were measured by air (250Hz to 16000Hz) and bone conduction (500Hz to 4000Hz). Then, acuphenometry was performed. It is a subjective measurement of tinnitus pitch and loudness, since it is not possible to objectively measure the intensity and frequency of the symptom.

Pitch corresponds to the sense of frequency and loudness to the sense of intensity of tinnitus reported by the patient. Patients were asked to compare their tinnitus to sounds emitted by the audiometer (pure tone or narrow band noise). [39] Acuphenometry was performed according to the procedure described by Branco-Barreiro. [40] Initially, pitch was measured. The hearing threshold of patients was selected in all frequencies, 10dBNA were added, and either pure tone or noise was presented, depending on patients' description of the characteristics of their tinnitus. Patients was asked to raise their hand when they realized that the sound they heard was similar to their tinnitus. After that, loudness was measured. The stimulus (pure tone or noise) was presented at the frequency indicated by the patient as similar to tinnitus, with initial intensity of 10dBNA below the patient's threshold. Then, intensity was increased 2dBNA at a time, and patients were asked to raise their hand at the time realized that the intensity presented was similar to that of their tinnitus. Such intensity was recorded and subtracted from the individual's hearing threshold. This calculation determined tinnitus loudness.

After that, the following measurements were performed: loudness discomfort levels, acoustic immitance, with tympanometry and contralateral and ipsilateral acoustic reflexes, transient evoked otoacoustic emissions and distortion product otoacoustic emissions. In specific situations, patients were evaluated for auditory evoked potentials.

After the completion of all tests, the subjects underwent medical evaluation again to determine the etiology and appropriate treatment for each case.

This study focuses on results of the evaluation of patients through acuphenometry, considering tinnitus pitch and loudness. Patients who had all assessments described above were included in the study.

The analysis was done by descriptive quantitative statistics, considering the absolute and relative values of the variables studied. The comparison of the results for THI between the groups used non-parametric tests (Mann-U-Whitney and Kruskal-Wallis), because the variable follows a non-normal distribution. To study the correlations between variables, the Spearman correlation coefficient was used.

Results

Examinations were evaluated for 199 patients seen at the chronic tinnitus outpatient clinic. According to data shown in Table 1, the highest prevalence was in females (62.3%), the mean age was 58.18 ± 12.79 years, with bilateral tinnitus (50.8%). The length of presence of the symptom ranged from less than one year to 32 years, with a mean time of 5.18 ± 4.67 years. Mean tinnitus pitch in both ears was approximately 4000Hz, while mean loudness was approximately 15dBNA. THI scores showed a mean of 40.03 ± 25.48. However, the analysis of grading by the instrument showed a greater number of individuals with slight, mild and moderate discomfort levels. In comparison, the grading of tinnitus severity, by the question about this, showed that subjects graded the discomfort caused by tinnitus between 2 and 10 points, averaging 5.18 ± 4.67 points.

Table 1. Descriptive analysis of the sample

Variables	**N**	**%**
Gender		
Male	75	62,3
Female	124	37,7
Age (years)		
Average ± standard deviation	58,18 ± 12,79	
Minimum - Maximum	19 - 82	
Time of tinnitus (years)		
Average ± standard deviation	5,18 ± 4,67	
Minimum - Maximum	0 – 32	
Location of tinnitus		
Right ear	47	23,6
Left ear	51	25,6
Both ears	101	50,8
Pitch of tinnitus (Hz)		
Right ear		
Average ± standard deviation	4359,80 ± 2735,54	
Minimum - Maximum	250 - 8000	
Left ear		
Average ± standard deviation	4458,88 ± 2678,63	
Minimum - Maximum	250 -9000	
Loudness of tinnitus (dB)		
Right ear		
Average ± standard deviation	16,65 ± 14,99	
Minimum - Maximum	0 -75	
Left ear		
Average ± standard deviation	15,84 ± 14,05	
Minimum - Maximum	0 - 70	
Score THI		
Average ± standard deviation	40,03 ± 25,48	
Minimum - Maximum	0 - 98	
Classification THI		
Slight	44	22,1
Mild	62	31,2

Table 1. (Continued)

Variables	N	%
Moderate	41	20,6
Severe	31	15,6
Catastrophic	21	10,6
Gravity of tinnitus		
Average ± standard deviation	5,18 ± 4,67	
Minimum - Maximum	2 - 10	

Correlation was analyzed between the variables THI score, age, tinnitus length, tinnitus severity, tinnitus pitch and tinnitus loudness (Table 2 and Table 3). There was a positive correlation between tinnitus severity and THI score ($r = 0.32$, $p < 0.001$) and negative and statistically significant correlations between age and THI score ($r = -0.254$, $p < 0.001$), and between age and tinnitus loudness in the left ear ($r = -0.18$, $p = 0.02$). There were no correlations between other variables: age and length of tinnitus ($r = 0.08$, $p = 0.24$), age and tinnitus severity ($r = 0.11$, $p = 0.11$), age and tinnitus pitch and tinnitus loudness in the right ear ($r = -0.03$, $p = 0.67$ and $r = -0.18$, $p = 0.29$, respectively), age and tinnitus pitch in the left ear (r = 0 , 02, $p = 0.80$), length of tinnitus and THI score ($r = 0.01$, $p = 0.78$), length of tinnitus presence and tinnitus severity ($r = -0.06$; $p = 0.38$), length of tinnitus presence and tinnitus pitch and loudness in the right ear ($r = -0.06$, $p = 0.43$ and $r = -0.24$, $p = 0.78$, respectively) and in the left ear (r = -, 014, $p = 0.06$ and $r = -0.33$, $p = 0.68$, respectively). Tinnitus severity was not associated with length of tinnitus presence ($r = -0.06$, $p = 0.38$), nor with tinnitus pitch and loudness in the right ear ($r = 0.00$, p = 0, 91 $r = -0.32$, $p = 0.70$, respectively) and in the left ear ($r = -0.49$, $p = 0.55$ and $r = 0.03$, $p = 0.63$, respectively).

Table 2. Analysis of the correlation between gender and scores on THI

	THI score			
	Average	**Median**	**Minimum**	**Maximum**
Female	40,3	36	0	98
Male	39,6	36	0	90

p-value – 0,82 (Mann-Whitney).

Table 3. Location of the THI score and tinnitus

	THI Score			
	Average	**Median**	**Minimum**	**Maximum**
Right ear	40,4	36	6	96
Left Ear	37,8	32	0	98
Both ears	41,0	36	0	90

p-value – 0,69 (Kruskal-Wallis).

Discussion

The results obtained in the study show that the sample was composed mostly by females. This finding is in disagreement with some studies that showed a similar number of men and women, [14] or a greater number of men,[17-19] but it is equivalent to others. [10, 15, 16] In the study group, women may be considered to be more affected by tinnitus, but the data may also reflect a situation that Brazilian women seek health services more often. [41, 42]

The age of the studied subjects ranged between 19 and 82 years, with a mean of 58.18 ± 12.79 years. It was found that 121 (60.80%) patients were younger than 65 years old, which is indicative that the sample consisted primarily of adults, similar to samples of other recent studies. [18,26] The lower presence of elderly in the sample was not expected by the researchers, since the literature reports an increase in the symptom with aging, [9] but it can be indicative of two possibilities. One is the decrease of the current age of individuals affected by tinnitus who seek specialized care. Another possibility to explain the age of treated patients is the association between tinnitus and resilience. Patients who complain about tinnitus and discomfort are seen in the outpatient clinic. It is known that elderly people have higher levels of resilience than adults, and that greater resilience is associated with less discomfort caused by tinnitus. A study on resilience showed that it is associated with better emotional health, which, in turn, stops tinnitus from having such a negative impact on quality of life. [23]

No children and adolescents were evaluated, although the technical literature reported that tinnitus can be observed in individuals of various age groups, and there is a high prevalence of children with the symptom. [12, 13] This can be explained by the fact that parents do not always know the complaints and otologic symptoms of their children, and the latter rarely report tinnitus spontaneously. [13] Thus, it is crucial for parents and health professionals who evaluate children to investigate the presence of tinnitus, so that etiology is clarified and appropriate treatment is given, since 19.6% of children may report discomfort by the presence of the symptom. [13]

The length of tinnitus presence in the subjects of the sample was 5.18 ± 4.67 years, similar to the results of one study conducted in the USA, whose sample was comprised of some Brazilian individuals. [26] Length, however, was lower than in other studies, [44-46] and most evaluated patients had bilateral tinnitus (50.8%), which is consistent with previous studies [46-48] but it is in disagreement with others, where there was a predominance of tinnitus in the left ear. [18, 26] It is believed that the results obtained in the present research, as regards tinnitus location, can be attributed to the etiology of the symptom, predominantly caused by presbycusis, noise-induced hearing loss and metabolic changes.

The study of psychoacoustic characteristics of tinnitus showed mean pitch of about 4000 Hz in both ears and mean loudness of 16.65 dB HL in the right ear and 15.84 dB HL in the left ear. The values were lower than in other studies. [45, 46] Previous studies showed an average tinnitus pitch of 6000 Hz and tinnitus loudness between 51dBNA and 61dBNA. This large difference in loudness can be explained by the evaluation method used in the studies.

THI scores ranged between 0 and 98 points, averaging 40.03 ± 25.48 points. The values were similar to those of another study. [46] The analysis of THI grading showed that most of the evaluated patients had mild discomfort (31.2%), followed by slight (22.1%) and moderate discomfort (20.6%).

The analysis of THI score and gender, and THI score and tinnitus location showed no significant differences. These data had already been described by other authors. [14, 48]

The analysis of the correlations between the characteristics of tinnitus, tinnitus discomfort and tinnitus severity showed that there was a positive correlation between tinnitus severity graded by patients and THI score. Thus, the higher the score on the scale, the greater the discomfort caused by tinnitus in the assessment made by THI. These data were expected by the researchers, since both tests evaluated the impact of tinnitus on patients' life. A similar result was obtained in a previous study which analyzed the relationship between the responses from THI and the visual analogue scale. [38]

There was also a negative and significant correlation between age and THI score, indicating that the higher the age, the lower the score. The analysis of these data and the fact that there was no correlation between age and most psychoacoustic characteristics of tinnitus (pith and loudness), seem to confirm that individuals adapt more easily to the symptom as they grow older. Again, resilience must be taken into account. [23] These data, however, differ from results of other studies that used the same instrument to assess the impact of tinnitus and found no relationship between age and THI score [18, 20,48, 49] or even an increase of the impact of tinnitus with increasing age. [47]

Conclusion

Data analysis has shown that the majority of the sample was comprised of female adults who had had tinnitus for about five years in both ears. Tinnitus pitch was acute and tinnitus loudness was moderate, within the values reported by the technical literature. The discomfort caused by tinnitus was mostly mild, slight or moderate, and subjects rated the discomfort caused by tinnitus as grade 5.

No difference was found between THI scores and gender and tinnitus location. There was correlation between severity of tinnitus and THI score, between age and tinnitus loudness in the left ear, and between age and THI score.

References

[1] Jastreboff PJ. Tinnitus retraining therapy. *Prog. Brain Res.*, 2007 166, 415-423.

[2] Baguley D; McFerran D; Hall D. Tinnitus. *Lancet*, 2013 382, 1600-1607.

[3] Fernandes G; Gonçalves DAG; Siqueira JTT; Camparis CM. Painful temporomandibular disorders, self reported tinnitus, and depression are highly associated. *Arq. Neuropsiquiatr.* 2013 71, 943-947.

[4] Landgrebe M; Zeman F; Koller M; Eberl Y; Mohr M; Reiter J; Staundinger S; Hajak G; Langguth B. The tinnitus research initiative (TRI) database: a new approach for delineation of tinnitus subtypes and generation of predictors for treatment outcome. *BMC Medical Informatics and Decision Making,* 2010 10, 42.

[5] Park KH; Lee SH; Koo J; Park HY; Lee KY; Choi YS; Oh KW; Lee A; Yang J; Woo SY; Kim SW; Choo YS. Prevalence and factors associated factors of tinnitus: data from

the Korean National Health and nutrition examination survey 2009-2011. *J. Epidemiol.,* 2014, 24, 417-426.
[6] Michikawa T; Nishiwaki Y; Kikuchi Y; Salto H; Mizutari K; Okamoto M; Takebayashi T. Prevalence and factors associated with tinnitus: a community-based study of Japanese elders. *J. Epidemiol.,* 2010 20, 271-276.
[7] Khedr EM; Ahmed MA; Shawky OA, Mohamed ES; El Atar GS; Mohammad KA. Epidemiological study of chronic tinnitus in Assiut, Egypt. *Neuroepidemiology,* 2010 35: 45-52.
[8] Shagorodsky J; Curhan CG; Farwell WR. Prevalence and characteristics of tinnitus among US adults. *Am. J. Med.*, 2010 123, 711-718.
[9] Jastreboff PJ; Hazzel JWP. A neurophysiological approach of tinnitus: clinical implications. *Br. J. Audiol.*, 1993 27,7-17.
[10] Carmo LC; Silveira JAM; Marone SAM; D'Ottaviano FG; Zagati LL; Lins EMDS. Audiological study of an elderly brazilian population. *Braz. J. Otorhinolaryngol.*, 2008, 74, 342-349.
[11] Coelho CCB; Sanchez TG; Bento RP. Caracterização do zumbido de pacientes atendidos em serviço de referência. *Arq. Int. Otorrinolaringol.*, 2004 8.
[12] Sanchez TG. "Epidemics" of tinnitus in the 21st century: preparing our children and grandchildren. *Braz. J. Otorhinolaringol.*, 2014 80, 3-4.
[13] Knobel KAB; Lima MCMP. Are parents aware of their children's hearing complaints? *Braz. J. Otorhinolaryngol.,* 2012 78, 27-37.
[14] Fioretti AB; Fusetti M; Eibenstein A. Association between sleep disorders, hyperacusis and tinnitus questionnaires. *Noise Health*, 2013 15, 91-95.
[15] Seydel C; Haupt H; Olze H; Szczepek AJ; Mazurek B. Gender and chronic tinnitus: differences in tinnitus-related distress depend on age and duration of tinnitus. *Ear hear*, 2013 34, 661-672.
[16] Lin Z; Qi M; Zeng X. Study on gender difference of tinnitus in medical staff. *Lin chung er bi yan hou tou jing wai ke za zhi*, 2013 27. 465-467.
[17] Teixeira AR; Nunes MGP; Freitas CLR; Gonçalves AK; Teixeira, SB. Analysis of quality of life of seniors with tinnitus' symptoms. *Intl. Arch. Otorhinolaryngol.*, 2010 14, 54-59.
[18] Udupi VA; Uppunda AK; Mohan KM; Alex J; Mahendra MH. The relationship of perceived severity of tinnitus with depression, anxiety, hearing status, age and gender in individuals with tinnitus. *Int. Tinnitus J.*, 2013 18, 29-34.
[19] Zeman F; Koller M; Langguth B; Landgrebe M. Which tinnitus-related aspects are relevant for quality of life and depression: results from a large international multicentre sample. *Health Qual. Life Outcomes*, 2014 12:7.
[20] Pinto PCL; Sanchez TG; Tomita S. The impacto of gender, age and hearing loss on tinnitus severity. *Braz. J. Otorhinolaryngol.*, 2010 76, 18-24
[21] Langguth B; Goodey R; Azevedo A; Bjorne A; Cacace A; Crocetti A; Vergara R. Consensus for tinnitus patient assessment and treatment outcome measurement: Tinnitus Research Initiative meeting. *Progress in brain research,* 2007 166: 525-536.
[22] Holgers KM; Zoger S; Svedlund K. Predictive factors for development of severe tinnitus suffering further characterization. *Int. J. Audiol.*, 2005 44, 584-592.

[23] Wallhäuser-Franke E; Delb W; Balkenhol T; Hiller W; Hörmann K. Tinnitus-related distress and the personality characteristic resilience. *Neural Plasticity,* 2014 article ID 370307, 6 pages.

[24] Geocze L; Mucci S; Abranches DC; Marco MA; Penido NO. Systematic review on the evidences of an association between tinnitus and depression. *Braz. J. Otorhinolaryngol.,* 2013 79, 106-111.

[25] Langguth B; Kleinjung T; Landgrebe M. Tinnitus: the complexity of standartization. *Eval. Health Prof.,* 2011 34: 429-433.

[26] Zeman F; Koller M; Scheklmann M; Langguth B; Landgrebe M. Tinnitus assessment by means of standartized self-reported questionnaires: psychometric properties of the Tinnitus Questionaire (TQ), the Tinnitus handicap Inventory (THI), and their short versions in an international multi-lingual sample. *Health Qual. Life Outcomes,* 2012 10:128.

[27] Kumral TL; Yldrm G; Yilmaz HB; Ulusoy S; Berkiten G; Onol SD; Ozturkçu Y; Uyar Y. Is it necessary to do temporal bone computed tomography of the internal auditory canal in tinnitus with normal hearing? *The Scientific World Journal,* 2013.

[28] Newman CW, Jacobson GP, Spritzer JB. Development of the Tinnitus Handicap Inventory. *Arch. Otolaryngol. Head Neck Surg.,* 1996 122, 143-148.

[29] Schimidt LP; Teixeira VN; Dall'Igna C; Dallagnol D; Smith MM. Brazilian Portuguese language version of th "Tinnitus Handicap Inventory": validity and reproducibility. *Braz. J. Otorhinolaryngol.,* 2006 72, 808-810.

[30] Meng Z; Zheng Y; Liu S; Wang K; Kong X; Tao Y; Xu K; Liu G. Reliability and validity of the Chinese (mandarin) tinnitus handicap inventory. *Clin. Exp. Otorhinolaryngol.,* 2012 5, 10-16.

[31] Kam AC; Cheung AP; Chan PY; Leung EK; Wong TK; van Hasselt CA; Tong MC. Psychometric properties of the Chinese (Cantonese) tinnitus handicap inventory. *Clin. Otolaryngol.,* 2009 34: 309-315.

[32] Ghulyan-Bédikian V; Paolino M; Giorgetti-D'Esclers F; Paolino F. Psychometric properties of a French adaptation of the tinnitus handicap inventory. *Encephale,* 2010 36, 390-396.

[33] Monzani D; Genovese E; Marrara A; Gherpelli C; Pingani L; Forghieri M; Rigatelli M; Guadagnin T; Arslan E. Validity of the Italian adaptation of the tinnitus handicap inventory; focus on quality of life and pdychological distress in tinnitus-sufferers. *Acta Otorrinolaryngol. Ital.,* 2008 28, 126-134.

[34] Der C; Alzérreca E; San Martín JT; Román L; Zamorano I; Malhue J; Aliaga P; Coronelli L; Sarda S. National linguistic validation of the tinnitus handicap inventory (THI). Assessment of disability caused by tinnitus in chilean spanish-speaking population. *Int. Tinnitus J.,* 2012 17, 146-151.

[35] Tobias CA; Llanes EG; Chiong C. Validity of a Filipino translation of the tinnitus handicap inventory. *Int. Tinnitus J.,* 2012 17: 64-69.

[36] Mahmoudian S; Shahmiri E; Rouzbahani M; Jafari Z; Keyhani M; Rahimi F; Mahmoudian G; Akbarvand L; Barzegar G; Farhadi M. Persian language version of the tinnitus handicap inventory: translation, standartization, validity and reliability. *Int .Tinnitus J.,* 2011 16: 93-103.

[37] Newman CW; Sandridge SA; Bolek L. Development and psychometric adequacy of the screening version of the tinnitus handicap inventory. *Otol. Neurotol.*, 2008 29: 276-281.

[38] Figueiredo RR; Azevedo AA; Oliveira PM. Correlation analysis of the visual-analogue scale and the Tinnitus Handicap Inventory in tinnitus patients. *Braz. J. Otorhinolaryngol.*, 2009 75, 76-79.
[39] Sanchez TG; Ferrari GMS. O que é zumbido? In: Samelli AG. *Zumbido – avaliação, diagnóstico e reabilitação.* São Paulo: Lovise, 2004.
[40] Branco-Barreiro FMA. Avaliação audiológica básica e psicoacústica do zumbido. In: In: Samelli AG. *Zumbido – avaliação, diagnóstico e reabilitação.* São Paulo: Lovise, 2004.
[41] Pinheiro RS; Viacava F; Travassos C; Brito AS. Gender, morbidity, access and utilization of health services in Brazil. *Ciência e Saúde Coletiva*, 2002 7, 687-707.
[42] Couto MT; Pinheiro TF; Valença O; Machin R; Silva GSN; Gomes R; Schraiber LB; Figueiredo WS. Men in primary healthcare: discussing (in)visibility based on gender perspectives. *Interface (Botucatu)*, 2010 14: 257-270.
[43] Coelho CB; Sanchez TG; Tyler RS. Tinnitus in children and associated risk factors. *Prog. Brain Res.*, 2007 166, 179-191.
[44] Dib GC; Kasse CA; Andrade TA; Testa JRG; Cruz OLM. Tinnitus treatment with tradozone. *Braz. J. Otorhinolaryngol.*, 2007 73, 390-397.
[45] Hoekstra CEL; Wesdorp FM; Zanten GA. Socio-demographic, health, and tinnitus related variables affecting tinnitus severity. *Ear Hear,* 2014 35, 544-554.
[46] Schecklmann M; Landgrebe M; Langguth B. Phenothypic characteristics of hyperacusis and tinnitus. *Plos. One,* 2014 9, e86944.
[47] Hiller W; Goebel G. Factors influencing tinnitus loudness and annoyance. *Arch. Otolaryngol. Head Neck Surg.*, 2006 132, 1323-1330.
[48] Mondelli MFCG; Rocha AB. Correlation between the audiologic findings and tinnitus disorder. *Intl. Arch. Otorhinolaryngol.,* 2011 15, 172-180.
[49] Milerová J; Anders M; Dvorak T; Sand PG; Königer S; Langguth B. The influence of psychological factors on tinnitus severity. *Gen. Hosp. Psychiatr.*, 2013 35, 412-416.

In: Handbook of Hearing Disorders Research
Editor: Charlotte Hailee Atkinson

ISBN: 978-1-63463-654-4

Chapter 6

The Molecular Pathogenesis of Dominant Deafness: Onychodystrophy (DDOD) Syndrome

Yongyi Yuan[1,2], Xi Lin[2] and Pu Dai[1]
[1]Department of Otolaryngology, Chinese PLA General Hospital, Beijing, People's Republic of China
[2]Department of Otolaryngology, Emory University School of Medicine, Atlanta, GA, US

Abstract

Dominant deafness-onychodystrophy syndrome (DDOD, MIM 124480) is a type of ectodermal dysplasia characterized mainly by congenital deafness, absent nails and/or toes with variable presence of brachydactyly, hypoplastic distal phalanges, and bulbous distal phalanges. Using the whole-exome sequencing approach, we identified a de novo mutation (c.1516 C>T [p.Arg506X]) in ATP6V1B2 as the cause of DDOD syndrome in three independently identified individuals. Molecular epidemiology analysis showed that the ATP6V1B2 p.Arg506X mutation was not present in 1053 ethnically matched normal hearing controls. ATP6V1B2 encodes a component of the vacuolar ATPase (V-ATPase, also known as H+-ATPase), a multisubunit enzyme that mediates acidification of eukaryotic intracellular organelles. We generated an Atp6v1b2 knockdown mouse model and found that Atp6v1b2 deficiency leads to severe sensorineural hearing loss. In vitro pathogenic evaluation showed that the ATP6V1B2 p.Arg506X mutation is a dominant haplo-insufficient mutation that caused abnormal acidification in the lysosomes. The acidification defect in lysosomes may cause decreased activity of acid-dependent hydrolases and thus hydrolytic dysfunction of the lysosome affects development of multiple systems such as the inner ear, phalanx, and nail in the DDOD syndrome. The findings provide the molecular basis for DDOD genetic diagnosis as well as exciting developments in future therapeutic interventions.

Introduction

Dominant deafness-onychodystrophy syndrome (DDOD syndrome, MIM 124480) is characterized mainly by congenital sensorineural hearing loss, and accompanied by dystrophic or absent nails. In some individuals, conical and hypoplastic teeth may also be observed. Prominent differences between DDOD and DOORS syndrome (deafness, onychodystrophy, osteodystrophy, intellectual disability and seizures, MIM 220500) are the intellectual disability and seizure aspects of DOORS [1]. *TBC1D24* mutations were verified as a cause of DOORS syndrome recently [2]. The association between deafness and onychodystrophy segregating as an autosomal dominant condition was first recognized in 1962 by Robinson et al. [3], and later was confirmed by Kondoh et al.[4] as well as White and Fahey [5]. To date, ten families with DDOD syndrome in various ethnic populations have been reported [2-9]. However, the molecular etiology of DDOD remains unknown. In this chapter, we report the identification of a common *de novo* mutation in *ATP6V1B2* among three independent Chinese families with the DDOD syndrome. We will present evidence supporting that *ATP6V1B2* is essential for hearing and that the identified mutation causes abnormal acidification in the lysosome.

Pedigrees and Clinical Evaluations

Three DDOD pedigrees were collected in China during the year 2011~2012. The DDOD pedigrees 1 and 3 were ascertained from Shanxi province, and pedigree 2 was from Jilin province of mainland China. The probands displayed identical phenotypes including severe congenital sensorineural hearing loss, absence of all toe nails, absence of nails on the little finger and thumb, phalanx deficiency of the little finger, onychodystrophy-like malacia, and pitting of the middle three fingernails (Figure 1). The gross inner ear structure was normal in all probands in this study as assessed by magnetic resonance imaging and high-resolution temporal bone computed tomography (Figure 1). All three individuals had unilateral cochlea implantation at the ages of 2.5, 2, and 18 years, respectively. Cognitive evaluation was performed using selected subclasses from a Chinese revised version of Griffiths Mental Development Scales (GMDS, 0-8 years of age) prior to cochlea implant operation[10]. The normal range of General Quotients of the Griffith test was above 70 in non-syndromic Chinese hearing loss individuals, and cases 1 and 2 scored 75 and 77, respectively. After cochlea implantation, language rehabilitation in the probands from pedigree 1 and pedigree 2 showed no distinct difference compared to other nonsyndromic hearing loss individuals. Although the proband in pedigree 3 had prelingual hearing loss and had received a cochlea implant as an adult, she made significant improvement in speech perception in both listening and pronunciation skills due to speech training in a language rehabilitation school from the age of 3 years. This successful language rehabilitation in the three DDOD probands further confirmed their normal mental development.

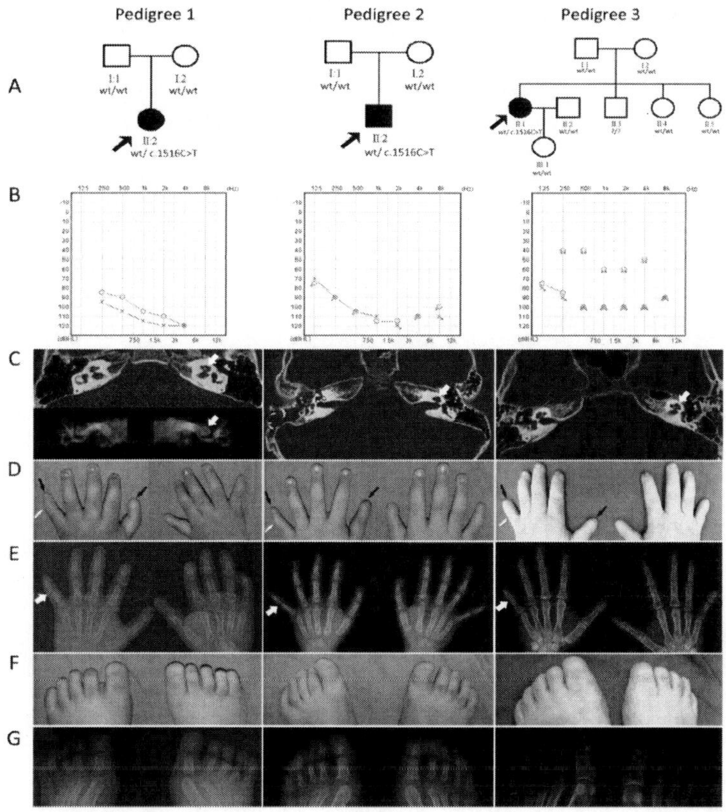

(A) Pedigree of three DDOD families and segregation of the c.1516 C>T mutation. The DNA sample of II:3 is not available in Pedigree 3.

(B) Audiograms of three probands showing bilateral severe sensorineural hearing loss. The blue curves indicate the left ear and red curves indicate the right ear.

(C) High resolution radiology results using computed tomography (CT) or magnetic resonance imaging (MRI) show normal inner ear development indicated by white arrows. Note: Due to infection of the first cochlear implant, the proband of Pedigree 2 received a second cochlear implant operation. The CT image shown here was obtained prior to implantation of the second cochlear implant. The implanted cochlea is indicated by the blue arrow.

(D) Pictures of the hands show the absence of the fifth finger and thumb nails indicated by black arrows, fifth finger phalanx deficiency indicated by white arrows, as well as onychodystrophy-like malacia and pitting of the middle three fingernails.

(E) X-ray of the hand shows fifth finger phalanx deficiency indicated by white arrows.

(F) Pictures of the feet show the absence of all toenails.

(G) X-ray of the foot shows no abnormalities.

Figure 1. Phenotype of the three Chinese DDOD (dominant deafness-onychodystrophy) probands.

Evidence Support that a De Novo Mutation in ATP6V1B2 Causes the DDOD Syndrome

Blood samples (~3-5 ml) were drawn from 6 participants so that genomic DNA could be extracted with the Genomic DNA isolation kit (QIAGEN). Paternity was confirmed by genotype analysis of 19 informative short tandem repeats (STRs) using Goldeneye™ 20A kit (Peoplespot, Beijing, China) [11], yielding a probability of paternity of 0.999999 (assuming a prior probability of 0.50). Exome capture was performed in pedigrees 1 and 2, including the two probands and their parents, by BGI–Shenzhen using NimbleGen SeqCap EZ Human Exome Library v2.0 (Roche NimbleGen, Inc., Madison, WI, USA) according to the manufacturer's protocols, and sequencing was performed using a HiSeq2000 platform (Illumina, San Diego, CA, USA). Illumina base calling Software 1.7 was used with default parameters to process the raw image files and to sequence the individual products as 90-bp paired-end reads. The sequenced reads were aligned to the human genome reference (UCSC hg19 version, build37.1) using SOAP aligner/SOAP2 [12]. SNP or indels were called using Soapsnp [13] software and bwa [14], respectively. The alignment results were identified using GATK [15] to identify the breakpoints.

In each sample, we obtained approximately 5.9–6.9 Gb of data after whole exome sequencing. The data mapped to the targeted region have a mean depth of 145.74 folds, and 99.41% of the targeted bases was covered. For bioinformatic analysis, we focused on variants in coding regions. Variants in individuals and their parents were filtered by four databases, including the 1000 Genomes Project, HapMap database, the EVS database, and in-house database from the BGI, with the Minor Allele Frequency lower than 0.005. Based on 1) the dominant inheritance of DDOD, 2) the identical phenotype of the two probands, and 3) the pedigree traits (only one individual and neither parent had symptoms) based on the assumption that there may be a de novo mutation following the dominant inheritance characteristics. Under assumptions of the autosomal-dominant analysis strategy (when incomplete penetrance can be excluded), the case must have a heterozygous mutation in a certain gene, while the control has no mutation. After completing such a filtering process, we identified 6 genes with variants shared by the two individuals (Table 1). Detailed variants in the six shared genes can be found in Table 2. Among the six genes, no known hearing-loss-related gene was identified. The 14 variants in the six shared genes were then tested by Sanger sequencing. Considering the sequencing results, the prediction results by SIFT, Polyphen, Mutationtaster, the genes' pathway and their expressions in human fetal cochlear ESTs database, *ATP6V1B2* was identified as the gene associated with DDOD. An identical heterozygous missense mutation (c.1516 C>T [p.Arg506X]) in *ATP6V1B2* was verified in two probands but not in their parents (Figure 2). The above results were further confirmed by Sanger sequencing in another DDOD pedigree (Pedigree 3) we collected in China, in which we found that the proband carried the same *ATP6V1B2* mutation. The *ATP6V1B2* c.1516 C>T (p.Arg506X) mutation segregated with the phenotype within the three DDOD families.

Table 1. Filtering of SNP variants obtained in whole exome NGS[9]

SNP Filter process	Individual 1	Individual 2
Total	110722	117704
Functional	14472	14642
Filtered_1000Genomes	2491	2545
Filtered_1000Genomes_Hapmap	2469	2521
Filtered_1000Genomes_Hapmap_EVS	2469	2521
Filtered_1000Genomes_Hapmap_EVS_control	215	242
Filtered_1000Genomes_Hapmap_EVS_control_BGI	83	96
Genes shared by individual 1 and individual 2	**6***	

* Details were shown in Table 2.

Table 2. Variants in the 6 genes shared by 2 DDOD cases [9]

	Gene Name	Codons	Substitution	Detailed Information for cases	Genotype Quality	Gene description
case 1	CIB1	-	-	W34A4T3,000, spliceAcceptorSite +6	Low_Confidence	calcium and integrin binding 1 (calmyrin)
	MUC4	CAC11271CAG	H3757Q	S99G123C9,000,missense	High_Confidence	mucin 4, cell surface associated
	MUC4	CCT4703CGT	P1568R	S41G191C7,000,missense	High_Confidence	mucin 4, cell surface associated
	OR5H6	ACT368CTT	T123L	Y97C23T9,000,missense	Low_Confidence	olfactory receptor, family 5, subfamily H, member 6
	PRAMEF1	ATG122AGG	M41R	K20T251G4,000,missense	High_Confidence	-
	AMBN	GGA539GTA	G180V	K43G137T9,000,missense	Low_Confidence	ameloblastin (enamel matrix protein)
	ATP6V1B2	CGA1516TGA	R506*	Y99T56C44,000,nonsense	High_Confidence	ATPase, H+ transporting, lysosomal 56/58kDa, V1 subunit B2
case 2	CIB1	-	-	W32T5A3,000,spliceAcceptorSite+6	Low_Confidence	calcium and integrin binding 1 (calmyrin)
	MUC4	CCT12574TCT	P4192S	R39G140A8,000,missense	High_Confidence	mucin 4, cell surface associated
	MUC4	ACC12568GCC	T4190A	Y45T119C7,000,missense	High_Confidence	mucin 4, cell surface associated
	MUC4	ATG4604ACG	M1535T	R22A54G5,000,missense	High_Confidence	mucin 4, cell surface associated
	OR5H6	GGG239GAG	G30E	R27G216A7,000,missense	High_Confidence	olfactory receptor, family 5, subfamily H, member 6

Table 2. (Continued)

	Gene Name	Codons	Substitution	Detailed Information for cases	Genotype Quality	Gene description
	PRAMEF1	ATG82GTG	M28V	R35A178G8,000,missense	High_Confidence	-
	AMBN	GGA539GCA	G180A	S22G129C6,000,missense	Low_Confidence	ameloblastin (enamel matrix protein)
	ATP6V1B2	CGA1516TGA	R506*	Y99T61C62,000,nonsense	High_Confidence	ATPase, H+ transporting, lysosomal 56/58kDa, V1 subunit B2

The p.Arg506X in *ATP6V1B2* is a nonsense mutation that inserts a premature stop codon, which results in a truncated protein that lacks the last five amino acids. Conservation analysis of amino acids in nine *ATP6V1B2* orthologs indicated that the last five amino acids (residues 506 to 511) are highly conserved (Figure 2). Three-dimensional protein structure modeling suggested that the p.Arg506X altered structure *of* ATP6V1B2, resulting in a failure of hydrogen bond formation between Tyr 504 and Asp 507 (Figure 3). The absence of this mutation in the parents of the three individuals indicates its *de novo* nature. Using a restriction enzyme (Taq I) assay to perform a molecular epidemiology analysis of the *ATP6V1B2* c.1516 C>T variation in 1053 ethnically matched normal hearing control subjects, we found that none of the normal hearing individuals showed such a mutation (Figure 4). In addition, the c.1516C>T variant is not seen in ESP65000 database.

Immunostaining of mouse cochlea sections and cultured cochlea tissues showed *Atp6v1b2* expression in the organ of Corti, spiral ganglion neurons, the limbus, and fibrocytes close to the stria vascularis (Figure 5). This expression pattern was found in both the early postnatal (postnatal day 2, orP2) and the adult (P30) cochleae.

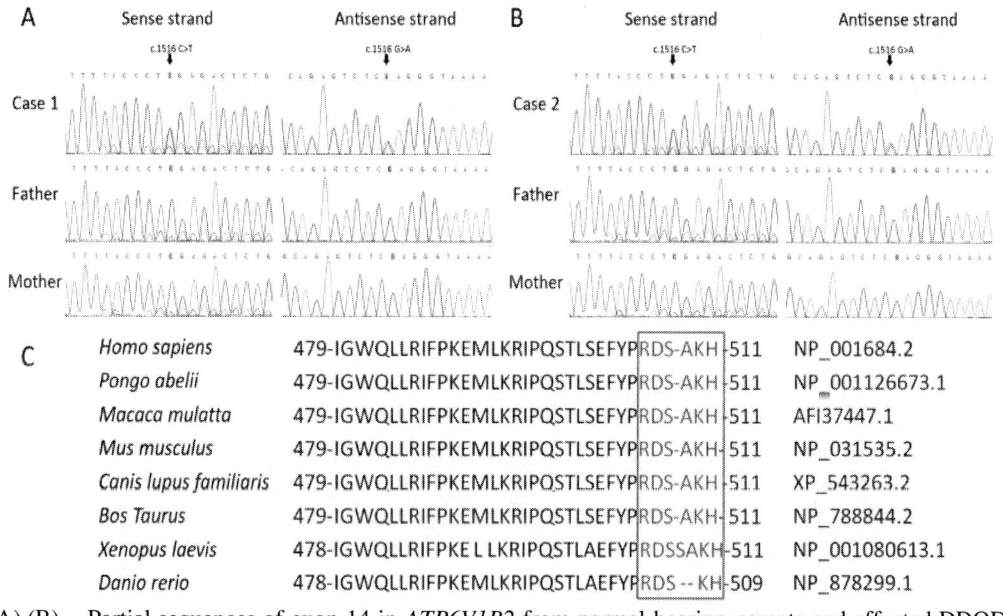

A),(B) Partial sequences of exon 14 in *ATP6V1B2* from normal-hearing parents and affected DDOD probands 1 and 2, respectively, showing the c.1516 C>T(p.Arg506X) nonsense mutation.

(C) Conservation analysis shows that the last six amino acids, p.Arg506, p.Asp507, p.Ser508, p.Ala509, p.Lys510 and p.His511 in ATP6V1B2 are conserved across human, pongo, macaca, mouse, canis, bos taurus, Xenopus and danio.

Figure 2. Mutation Analysis of ATP6V1B2.

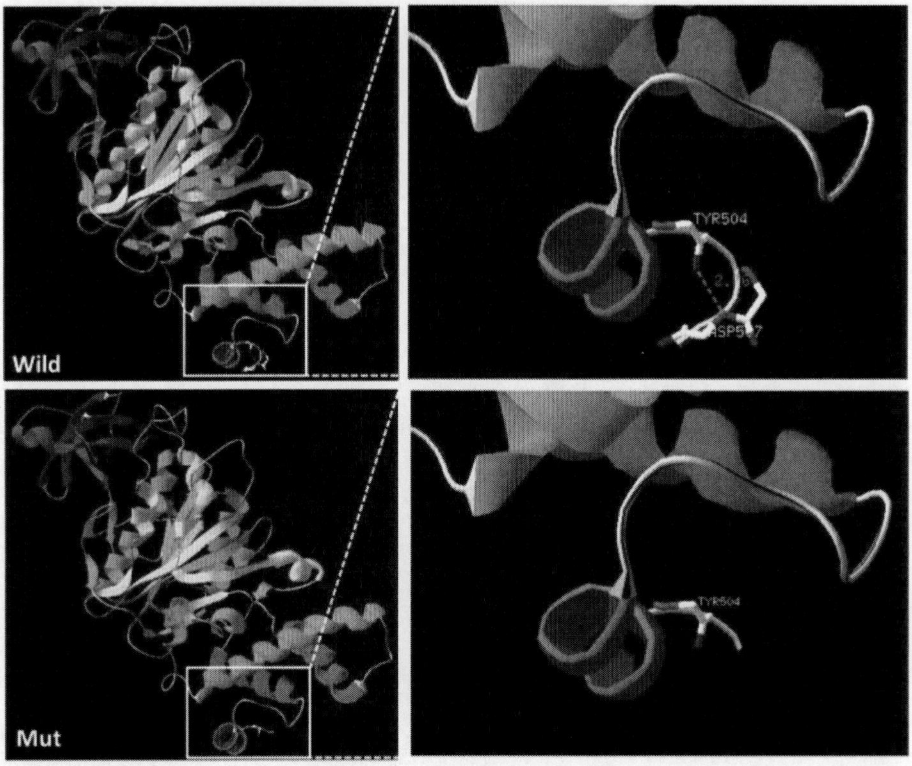

Structure analysis of the wild-type ATP6V1B2 and mutant ATP6V1B2 (by Swiss model Workspace: http://swissmodel.expasy.org/workspace/). p.Arg506X results in failure of hydrogen bond formation between Tyr 504 and Asp in ATP6V1B2.

Figure 3. Altered protein structure by *ATP6V1B2* p.Arg506X.

Example gel showing that three bands, 252bp, 165bp and 87bp, in individual with heterozygous *ATP6V1B2* c.1516 C>T mutation, and two bands, 165bp and 87bp, in wild-type controls. The pair of primers used for restriction enzyme reaction was designed around *ATP6V1B2* c.1516 C, which can amplify a fragment of 252bp. The restriction enzyme Taq I recognizes the 'TC' at c.1515 and c.1516. After the Taq I reaction, the 252bp fragment is cut into two fragments of 165 and 87 bp. However, the mutation c.1516 C>T deletes the Taq I restriction endonuclease site. Thus, for the heterozygous c.1516 C>T mutation, three bands (252, 165 and 87 bp) were detected, while in controls lacking the c.1516 C>T mutation, two bands (165 and 87 bp) were detected.

Figure 4. Taq I restriction enzyme assay showing normal versus ATP6V1B2 c.1516 C>T mutant PCR fragments.

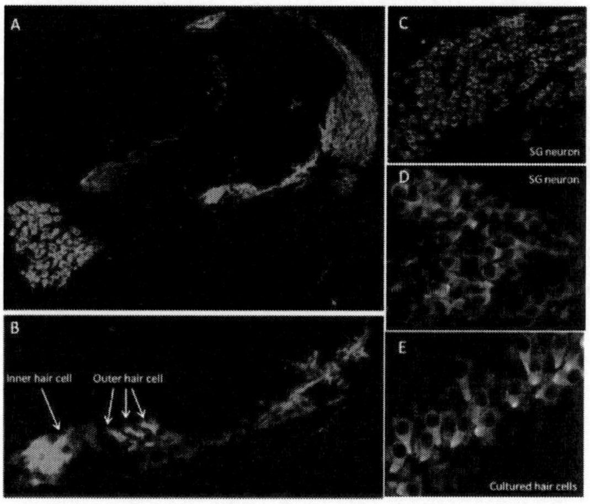

(A) Atp6v1b2 distribution in mouse cochlea. Atp6v1b2 expresses mainly in the organ of Corti, spiral ganglion neurons, the limbus, and fibrocytes close to the stria vascularis; (B) Atp6v1b2 expression in hair cells; (C) Atp6v1b2 expression in the spiral ganglia (SG) neurons; (D) Double staining of Atp6v1b2 and tubulin in ganglia neurons. Green: Atp6v1b2, Red: ß-tubulin; (E) Double staining of Atp6v1b2 and Myo6 in cultured hair cells. Green: Atp6v1b2, Red: Myo6

Figure 5. *Atp6v1b2* expression in the cochlea.

Atp6v1b2 Cochlea Knockdown Mouse Shows Hearing Loss

To further investigate the function of *ATP6V1B2* in the cochlea, we generated a mouse model in which the expression of Atp6v1b2 was specifically reduced in the cochlea using a morpholino oligomer. The oligomer was designed to anneal at the junction of intron 12 and exon 13, which resulted in a partial inclusion of intron 12 followed by a stop codon that excluded the expression of exons 13 and 14 in the mature mRNA (Figure 6A). The *Atp6v1b2* morpholino oligomer was microinjected (0.05–5.0 µg/µL) into the scala media of the basal turn of the mouse cochlea before postnatal day three. Hearing sensitivity has been shown to be unaffected by such an injection procedure if the injection was done to mice younger than postnatal day 5 (P5) [16]. Reverse transcription-polymerase chain reaction (RT-PCR) was used to verify the abnormal transcript product containing part of intron 12 in the mouse cochlea 3 days after injection (Figure 6A). At 4 weeks post-injection, auditory brainstem response (ABR) tests measured across a frequency range of 4–32 kHz showed that hearing thresholds in the ear injected with the morpholino oligomer at the concentration of 0.5, 1.25, 2.5 and 5.0 µg/µL were elevated by 30–50 dB compared to wild-type mice. However, hearing thresholds in mice injected with 0.05 µg/µL morpholino oligomer was within the normal range, indicating the dosage dependence of the hearing loss phenotype. In addition, all the mice received scrambled morpholino oligomer (0.5 µg/µL) displayed normal hearing (Figure 6B). These results supported the specific effects of the injected morpholino oligomer. Immunological staining observations revealed that *Atp6v1b2* expression was knocked down significantly in the gross cochlea (Figure 7), especially in the hair cells and the spiral ganglion neurons. In addition, we observed hair cell degeneration in the cochlea that received the morpholino oligomer to knockdown the *Atp6v1b2* expression (Figure 6C).

Western Blot Analysis of Atp6v1b2 Shows Reduced Expression of atp6v1b2 in the Spiral Ganglion Neurons and the Organ of Corti

Western blot analysis performed 7 days after injections demonstrated significantly decreased levels of V-ATPase encoded by *Atp6v1b2* in the group that received morpholino oligomer in both the spiral ganglion neurons (Tukey's multiple comparison test, *P*=0.0073, q=25.99) and in the organ of Corti. The comparsion was made between the experimental group and the group that received scrambled morpholino oligomer as well as the wild-type group. At three weeks after morpholino oligomer injection, the V-ATPase level was decreased further in the organ of Corti (Tukey's Test, *P*=0.039, q=10.37, Figure 8).

ATP6V1B2 C.1516 C>T is a Dominant Loss-of-Function Mutation, Causing Abnormal Acidification in Lysosomes

To evaluate the pathogenicity of the *ATP6V1B2* c.1516 C>T mutation, we transfected the pIRES2-EGFP-*ATP6V1B2* wild-type plasmid and pIRES2-EGFP-*ATP6V1B2* c.1516 C>T mutant plasmid into HEK293 cells. V-ATPase is expressed in HEK293 cells, and transfection with *ATP6V1B2* caused an overexpression of the V-ATPase. However, no change in *ATP6V1B2* intracellular distribution was detected in c.1516 C>T mutant-transfected cells. We found that the ATPase hydrolysis activity significantly decreased in the transfected cells when the ratio of the mutant increased. The ATPase hydrolysis in cells transfected with *ATP6V1B2* was 42.24 ± 2.11, that in cells transfected with a 1:1 mixture of *ATP6V1B2* and the c.1516 C>T mutant was 38.48 ± 2.87, and that in cells transfected with c.1516 C>T mutant was 36.09 ± 2.89. The ATPase hydrolysis activity in cells transfected with empty vector was 30.28 ± 2.79 (Newman-Keuls Multiple Comparison Test, *P*=0.032,q=4.508, Figure 9A). This trends indicated the c.1516 C>T mutant had reduced ATPase hydrolysis compared with the wild-type ATP6V1B2.

We measured the proton transport activity of V-ATPase in lysosomes using a lysosome-specific dye. The lysosome pH measurements were 5.02 ± 0.05 in cells transfected with empty vector control, 4.72 ± 0.046 in cells transfected with the c.1516 C>T mutant, 4.65 ± 0.042 in cells transfected with a 1:1 mixture of *ATP6V1B2* and the c.1516 C>T mutant, and 4.59 ± 0.048 in cells transfected with wild-type *ATP6V1B2.* A statistically significant difference in lysosomal pH was detected between *ATP6V1B2* and c.1516 C>T mutant-transfected cells (LSD test, *P*=0.02, Figure 9B and 9C). The ATPase hydrolysis activity and proton transport activity did not differ significantly between HEK293 cells and pIRES2-EGFP-transfected HEK293 cells. These results of the c.1516 C>T mutant that the V-ATPase hydrolysis decreased and the lysosome pH increased which indicated the reduced acidification suggest that *ATP6V1B2* c.1516 C>T is a loss-of-function mutation.

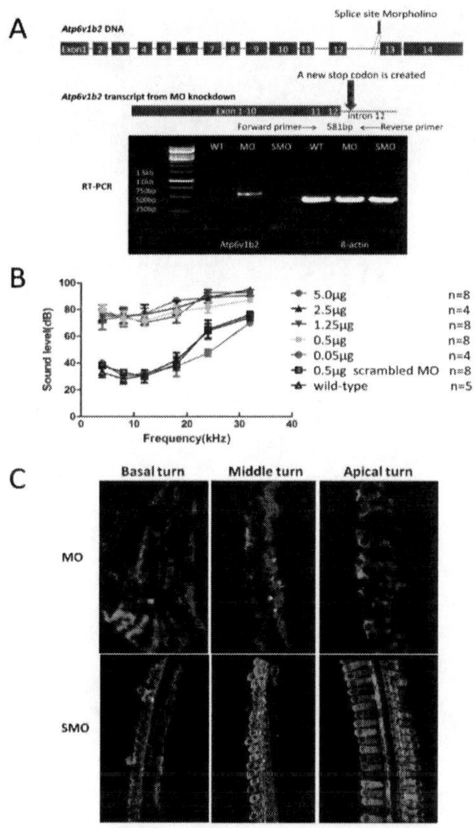

(A) RT-PCR analysis shows intron 12 retention in the *Atp6v1b2* transcript of *Atp6v1b2*-specific morpholino oligomer (MO)-knockdown mouse cochlea. The morpholino oligomer was designed to anneal at the junction of intron 12 and exon 13, which resulted in a partial inclusion of intron 12 followed by a stop codon UAA (indicated by the red arrow). The forward RT-PCR primer was in exon 11 and the reverse primer was in intron 12. The RNA was extracted 3 days after morpholino inner ear injection. Since the reverse primer corresponded to intron 12 sequences, it could not bind to the normal *Atp6v1b2* transcript. No bands were observed in the wild-type (WT)- or scrambled morpholino oligomer (SMO)-injected mice. The primer pairs amplified a product of 581 bp, including part of exon 11, exon 12 and part of intron 12 in the presence of abnormal splicing due to the *Atp6v1b2*-specific morpholino.

(B) Hearing thresholds (y-axis) were determined based on ABR measurements at various frequencies (x-axis) for *Atp6v1b2*-specific morpholino oligomer (MO)-knockdown mice, scrambled morpholino oligomer (SMO) control mice and wild-type mice. ABR thresholds were measured at postnatal day 30 (P30), 4 weeks after cochlea injection. Hearing thresholds in *Atp6v1b2*-knockdown mice at 0.5, 1.25, 2.5 and 5.0 μg/μL were elevated by ~30–50 dB compared with wild-type and scrambled-morpholino-injected mice. Hearing thresholds in *Atp6v1b2*-specific-MO-cochlea-injected mice at 0.05 μg/μL were within the normal range. Legends for different mouse groups are shown in the panel, n= the number of ears. Vertical bars represent standard errors of the mean.

(C) Flattened whole mount cochlea staining shows the degeneration of hair cells in the *Atp6v1b2*-knockdown mice. At 21 days after cochlea injection with *Atp6v1b2*-specific morpholino oligomer (MO, 0.5 μg), the majority of hair cells in the basal, middle, and apical turns had died. At 21 days after cochlea injection with the scrambled morpholino oligomer (SMO, 0.5 μg), the hair cells in the basal, middle and apical turns remained normal. Green: Atp6v1b2; Red: Phalloidin.

Figure 6. *Atp6v1b2*-knockdown analysis in the mouse cochlea.

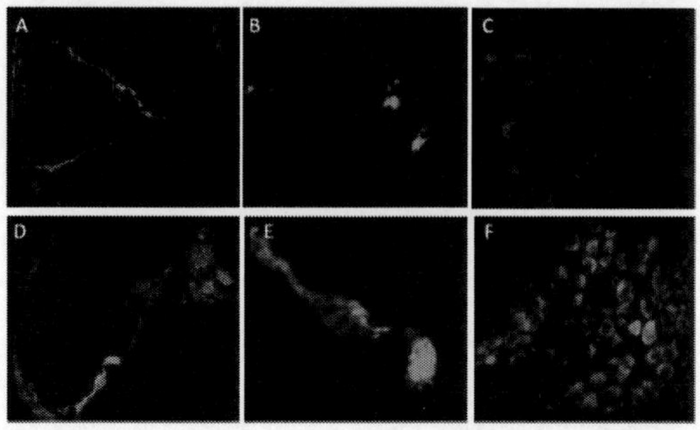

(A) Knockdown of *Atp6v1b2* in the whole cochlea 30 days after cochlea injection with *Atp6v1b2*-specific morpholino (0.5 μg); (B) Hair cell degeneration 30 days after cochlea injection with *Atp6v1b2*-specific morpholino (0.5 μg); (C) Spiral ganglia neuron degeneration 30 days after cochlea injection with *Atp6v1b2*-specific morpholino (0.5 μg); (D) to (F) Whole cochlea, hair cells and spiral ganglia neurons remain normal 30 days after cochlea injection with scrambled morpholino (0.5 μg). Green: Atp6v1b2

Figure 7. Degeneration of mouse spiral ganglia neurons and organ of Corti in *Atp6v1b2* knockdown mice.

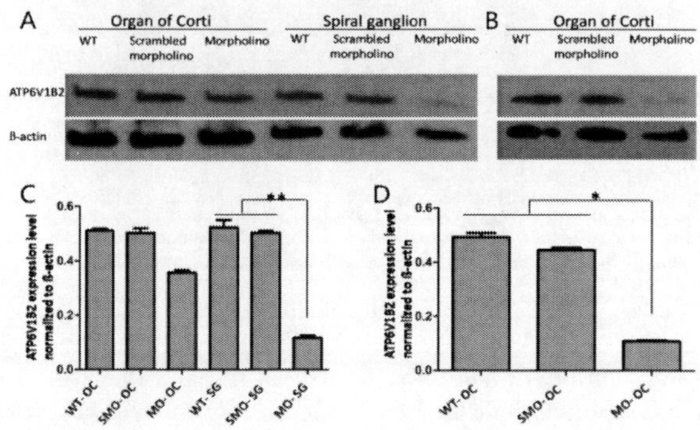

(A) Western blots of ATP6V1B2 in the organ of Corti (OC) and spiral ganglion (SG) of wild-type (WT), scrambled-morpholino-oligomer (SMO, 0.5 μg/μl) control and Atp6v1b2-specific morpholino oligomer (MO, 0.5 μg/μl)-knockdown mice. Legends for each lane are shown in the figure. Protein was extracted from the postnatal day 9 (P9) mouse cochlea 7 days after inner ear injection.

(B) Western blots of ATP6V1B2 in the organ of Corti (OC) of wild-type (WT), scrambled-morpholino-oligomer (SMO, 0.5 μg/μl) control and Atp6v1b2-specific-morpholino-oligomer (MO, 0.5 μg/μl)-knockdown mice. Legends for each lane are shown in the figure. Protein was extracted from postnatal day 23 (P23) mouse, 21 days after inner ear injection.

(C) The band intensities in Figure 8A were normalized to the corresponding ß-actin bands for quantification. Two asterisks on top of bars indicate significant reductions in ATP6V1B2 expression compared with the WT and SMO control in the spiral ganglion (Tukey's multiple comparison test, $P<0.01$). Data are presented as means ± standard deviation. Four biological replicates are represented in the bar graphs.

(D) The band intensities in Figure 8B were normalized to the corresponding ß-actin bands for quantification. The asterisk on top of the bars indicates significant reductions in ATP6V1B2 protein expression compared with the WT and SMO control in the organ of Corti (Tukey's multiple comparison test, $P<0.05$). Data are presented as means ± standard deviation. Four biological replicates are represented in the bar graphs.

Figure 8. Protein levels of ATP6V1B2 in two regions of the cochlea from wild-type, scrambled-morpholino-control and *Atp6v1b2*-knockdown mice.

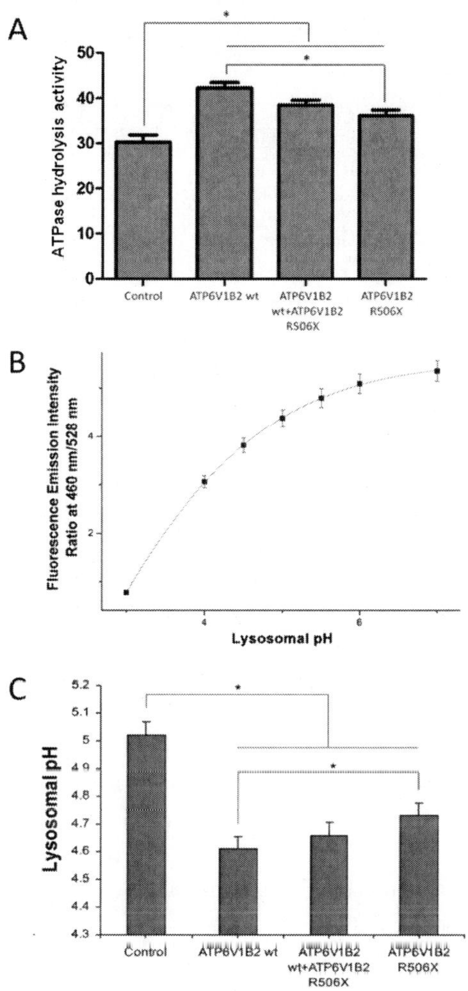

(A) ATPase assays showed that ATPase hydrolysis activity decreased significantly in the transfected cells as the ratio of the mutant increased. The data in each group represent a sample size (n) of 9. The asterisk on the top of bars indicates a significant increase or reduction in ATPase hydrolysis activity ($P<0.05$), compared to the empty vector control pIRES2-EGFP or pIRES2-EGFP-*ATP6V1B2,* respectively. Statistical analyses were performed by the Newman-Keuls Multiple Comparison Test. Data are presented as means ± standard deviation.

(B) Calibration curve for determining the lysosomal pH in HEK 293 cells. Calibration was performed as described in the Materials and Methods to generate a curve relating to the emission intensity ratio at 460 and 528 nm using an excitation at 360 nm to lysosomal pH. Vertical bars represent standard errors of the mean of four identical samples.

(C) The lysosomal pH increased in transfected cells as the ratio of the mutant increased, indicating that ATPase proton transport activity decreased as the ratio of the mutant increased. The data in each group represent a sample size (n) of 4. The asterisk on top of bars indicates significant reduction or increase in lysosomal pH ($P<0.05$), compared to the empty vector control pIRES2-EGFP or pIRES2-EGFP-*ATP6V1B2*, respectively. Statistical analyses were performed using the LSD Test. Data are presented as means ± standard deviation.

Figure 9. Effects of the ATP6V1B2 $^{p.Arg506X}$ mutant on ATPase activity in transfected HEK293 cells.

Discussion

Deafness and onychodystrophy diseases (DODs) are classified into two genetically distinct groups: the autosomal recessive form (DOOR syndrome) and the dominant (D) form (DDOD). Clinically, individuals with DOOR syndrome show features such as mild to severe mental retardation, seizures, mutism, hypotonia, congenital sensorineural deafness, triphalangeal thumbs, and hypoplastic nails. The phenotypes of DDOD are milder than those in the recessive form [3], and do not usually involve mental retardation. Features in our DDOD families resembled those reported in several previous studies [4-8] and included deafness, absence of nails and/or toes with more variable presence of brachydactyly, hypoplastic distal phalanges, and bulbous distal phalanges. Of note, the probands reported by Feinmesser and Zelig [8] were affected sisters from a consanguineous family; both had normal intellect, which was suggestive of autosomal recessive inheritance, genetic heterogeneity, or possibly gonadal mosaicism for an autosomal dominant condition. The conditions in the other reported families segregated in an autosomal dominant manner. To date, the hereditary pathogenesis has not been clarified for either DDOD or DOOR syndrome [1], although a neurometabolic etiology has been postulated for latter.

Prior to our study, White and Fahey [5] performed an SNP microarray analysis of one DDOD individual from Australia. However, they found no evidence of a change in copy number. Our study is the first report of a *de novo* heterozygous mutation in the *ATP6V1B2* gene that appeared to be a cause of autosomal DDOD syndrome. The *ATP6V1B2* gene on chromosome 8p21.3 contains 14 exons and normally encodes 511 amino acids. The availability of two independent individuals with a strikingly similar phenotype was very useful for identifying the causative gene and we took advantage of it. Our results obtained from these two individuals indicated that the *ATP6V1B2* defect causes DDOD syndrome, and this was further verified in a third independent family. The identification of the specific *ATP6V1B2* c.1516 C>T (p.Arg506X) mutation in three independently identified DDOD individuals, but not in a large number (1053 cases) of normal hearing controls, provides further supporting evidence that the p.Arg506X in *ATP6V1B2* is responsible for the DDOD syndrome.

Schinzel-Giedion syndrome (MIM 269150) and Kabuki syndrome (MIM 147920) [17,18] are known to be caused by dominant *de novo* mutations. D*e novo* mutations have recently been shown to play a major role in human diseases with reduced reproductive fitness [18-21]. The identification of a same *de novo* dominant mutation in 3 unrelated DDOD individuals by chance should be extremely unlikely. Our results indicate a high correlation between phenotype and genotype in these individuals with the DDOD syndrome. Given a transmission risk of 50% and a recurrence risk of <1% for *de novo* autosomal dominant mutations, compared to a transmission risk of <1% and a recurrence risk of 25% for autosomal recessive inheritance, the relatively high frequency of the *de novo* mutation in our cohort has significant implications for genetic counseling in our individuals and their relatives.

ATP6V1B2 encodes a component of the vacuolar ATPase (V-ATPase, also known as H+-ATPase), which is a multisubunit enzyme that mediates acidification of eukaryotic intracellular organelles. V-ATPase-dependent organelle acidification is necessary for intracellular processes such as protein sorting, zymogen activation, receptor-mediated endocytosis, and synaptic vesicle proton gradient generation. V-ATPase is composed of a cytosolic V1 domain and a transmembrane V0 domain. The V1 domain is responsible for ATP hydrolysis, and the V0 domain is responsible for protein translocation. The protein encoded by *ATP6V1B2* is one of the two V1 domain B subunit isoforms, and as it is highly expressed in the organ of cerebrum and in the organelle of *Atp6v1b2*, it is usually called a brain isoform or lysosomal V1 subunit B2 [22,23]. Deficiency in *ATP6V1B2* has been related to hereditary diseases such as osteopetrosis and renal tubular acidosis. It has been suggested that deficiencies of *ATP6V1B1* and *ATPV0A4* is related to distal renal tubular acidosis and hearing loss [24–27]. To the best of our knowledge, no report has linked the function of *ATP6V1B2* to hearing. The distribution of *Atp6v1b2* in hair cells and spiral ganglia neurons in mouse indicates it may play a role in the auditory system. The gene *related to* DOORS syndrome, *TBC1D24, encodes a member of the Tre2–Bub2–Cdc16 (TBC) domain-containing Rab (Ras-related proteins in brain)-specific GTPase-activating proteins, which coordinate Rab proteins and other GTPases for the regulation of membrane trafficking.* TBC1D24 and ATP6V1B2 are all known to be widely expressed, most highly in the brain and kidneys. *Tbc1d24* expresses in the stereocilia of the hair cells as well as in the spiral ganglion neurons [28]. TBC1D24 and ATP6V1B2's identical distribution regions and their function with GTPases or ATPases indicate they may have some physiological link. The hearing loss phenotype of our *Atp6v1b2* cochlea knockdown mouse model confirmed that the normal function of the gene is required for normal hearing. Significantly reduced *Atp6v1b2* expression in the mouse cochlea resulted in the death of hair cells and spiral ganglion neurons, leading to hearing loss.

Cell metabolism depends on the endocytic pathway [29,30]. Lysosomes, the terminal organelles in the endocytic pathway, play an important role in hydrolyzing macromolecules and making their components available as nutrients for the cell. Hydrolytic enzymes in lysosomes are activated by the acidic pH (between 4.5 and 5.0), which is generated and maintained by the activity of the proton-pumping V-ATPase, using metabolic energy in the form of ATP to pump protons into the lysosome lumen [31,32]. Our functional studies demonstrating that the c.1516 C>T mutation caused a decrease in the ATP production and an increase in lysosomal pH indicate that *ATP6V1B2* c.1516C>T is a dominant loss-of-function mutation. According to PhyloP vertebrate conservation scores, the *ATP6V1B2 c.*1516 C is a highly conserved base in the genome. The coded amino acid 506 is highly conserved according to multiple sequence alignment and mutant protein structure abnormality predicted by SWISS-MODEL [33]. These support the pathogenicity of the mutation. We propose that insufficient acidification in the lysosome caused by *ATP6V1B2* c.1516 C>T mutation may result in decreased activity of acid-dependent hydrolases, thereby limiting the decomposition of proteins, lipids, and polysaccharides in cells and affecting the development of multiple ectoderm-derived systems. Embryologically, the inner ear, nails, and teeth are all ectoderm-derived organs. The fact that *ATP6V1B2* is ubiquitously expressed in humans makes it reasonable to assume that *ATP6V1B2* may play important roles in other developing ectoderm-derived organs. Knock-in mouse model studies are underway in our laboratory to elucidate the consequences of *ATP6V1B2* mutation on ectoderm-derived organs, with the goal of targeting these effects therapeutically.

In summary, whole-exome sequencing in DDOD pedigrees revealed a *de novo* c.1516 C>T (p.Arg506X) mutation in *ATP6V1B2* that was present in three independently identified individuals with DDOD. Immunolabeling for localization of *ATP6V1B2* in the mouse cochlea as well as functional and morphological studies in the *ATP6V1B2* knockdown mouse model provided further evidences that support the idea that *ATP6V1B2* is a syndromic deafness gene. Direct assessment of the *in vitro* effects of the *ATP6V1B2* c.1516 C>T mutation in transfected cells indicated that it is a dominant haplo-insufficient mutation leading to insufficient acidification of the lysosome. Understanding molecular mechanisms in rare syndromic hearing impairments might lead to valuable insights into the molecular triggers for hair cell and spiral ganglion neuron degeneration and provide the basis for genetic diagnosis as well as new developments in future therapeutic interventions.

References

[1] James, A. W., Miranda, S. G., Culver, K., Hall, B. D. & Golabi, M. (2007). DOOR syndrome: clinical report, literature review and discussion of natural history. *Am J Med Genet A*, *143A*, 2821-2831.

[2] Vind-Kezunovic, D. & Torring, P. M. (2013). A Danish family with dominant deafness-onychodystrophy syndrome. *Journal of dermatological case reports*, *7*, 125-128.

[3] Robinson, G. C., Miller, J. R. & Bensimon, J. R. (1962). Familial ectodermal dysplasia with sensorineural deafness and other anomalies. *Pediatrics*, *30*, 797-802.

[4] Kondoh, T., Tsuru, A., Matsumoto, T., Matsuzaka, T. & Tsuji, Y. (1999). Autosomal dominant onychodystrophy and congenital sensorineural deafness. *J Hum Genet*, *44*, 60-62.

[5] White, S. M. & Fahey, M. (2011). Report of a further family with dominant deafness-onychodystrophy (DDOD) syndrome. *Am J Med Genet A*, *155A*, 2512-2515.

[6] Moghadam, H. & Statten, P. (1972). Hereditary sensorineural hearing loss associated with onychodystrophy and digital malformations. *Can Med Assoc J*, *107*, 310-312.

[7] Goodman, R. M., Lockareff, S. & Gwinup, G. (1969). Hereditary congenital deafness with onychodystrophy. *Arch Otolaryngol*, *90*, 474-477.

[8] Feinmesser, M. & Zelig, S. (1961). Congenital deafness associated with onychodystrophy. *Arch Otolaryngol*, *74*, 507-508.

[9] Yuan, *Y*., Zhang, *J*, Chang, Q., Zeng, J., Xin, F., et al. (2014). De novo mutation in ATP6V1B2 impairs lysosome acidification and causes dominant deafness-onychodystrophy syndrome. Cell research 10.1038/cr.2014.77.

[10] Wang, H. Q. *ea* (2007). Standardization of the Griffith Mental Development Scales for Children Aged 0~ 7 Years in the C ities of Shanxi Province. *Chinese Mental Health Journal*, *121*, 700-703.

[11] Tong, D., Chen, Y., Ou, X., Chen, W., Liu, S., et al. (2013). Polymorphism analysis and evaluation of 19 STR loci in the Han population of Southern China. *Ann Hum Biol*, *40*, 191-196.

[12] Li, R., Yu, C., Li, Y., Lam, T. W., Yiu, S. M., et al. (2009). SOAP2: an improved ultrafast tool for short read alignment. *Bioinformatics*, *25*, 1966-1967.

[13] Li, R., Li, Y., Fang, X., Yang, H., Wang, J., et al. (2009). SNP detection for massively parallel whole-genome resequencing. *Genome Res*, *19*, 1124-1132.

[14] Li, H. & Durbin, R. (2010). Fast and accurate long-read alignment with Burrows-Wheeler transform. *Bioinformatics*, *26*, 589-595.

[15] McKenna, A., Hanna, M., Banks, E., Sivachenko, A., Cibulskis, K., et al. (2010). The Genome Analysis Toolkit: a MapReduce framework for analyzing next-generation DNA sequencing data. *Genome Res*, *20*, 1297-1303.

[16] Wang, Y., Sun, Y., Chang, Q., Ahmad, S., Zhou, B., et al. (2013). Early postnatal virus inoculation into the scala media achieved extensive expression of exogenous green fluorescent protein in the inner ear and preserved auditory brainstem response thresholds. *J Gene Med*, *15*, 123-133.

[17] Ng, S. B., Bigham, A. W., Buckingham, K. J., Hannibal, M. C., McMillin, M. J., et al. (2010). Exome sequencing identifies MLL2 mutations as a cause of Kabuki syndrome. *Nat Genet*, *42*, 790-793.

[18] Hoischen, A., van Bon, B. W., Gilissen, C., Arts, P., van Lier, B., et al. (2010). De novo mutations of SETBP1 cause Schinzel-Giedion syndrome. *Nat Genet*, *42*, 483-485.

[19] Vissers, L. E., de Ligt, J., Gilissen, C., Janssen, I., Steehouwer, M., et al. (2010). A de novo paradigm for mental retardation. *Nat Genet*, *42*, 1109-1112.

[20] Vadlamudi, L., Dibbens, L. M., Lawrence, K. M., Iona, X., McMahon, J. M., et al. (2010). Timing of de novo mutagenesis--a twin study of sodium-channel mutations. *N Engl J Med*, *363*, 1335-1340.

[21] Hamdan, F. F., Gauthier, J., Spiegelman, D., Noreau, A., Yang, Y., et al. (2009). Mutations in SYNGAP1 in autosomal nonsyndromic mental retardation. *N Engl J Med*, *360*, 599-605.

[22] Wagner, C. A., Finberg, K. E., Breton, S., Marshansky, V., Brown, D., et al. (2004). Renal vacuolar H+-ATPase. *Physiol Rev*, *84*, 1263-1314.

[23] Nelson, N., Perzov, N., Cohen, A., Hagai, K., Padler, V., et al. (2000). The cellular biology of proton-motive force generation by V-ATPases. *J Exp Biol*, *203*, 89-95.

[24] Stover, E. H., Borthwick, K. J., Bavalia, C., Eady, N., Fritz, D. M., et al. (2002). Novel ATP6V1B1 and ATP6V0A4 mutations in autosomal recessive distal renal tubular acidosis with new evidence for hearing loss. *J Med Genet*, *39*, 796-803.

[25] Stehberger, P. A., Schulz, N., Finberg, K. E., Karet, F. E., Giebisch, G., et al. (2003). Localization and regulation of the ATP6V0A4 (a4) vacuolar H+-ATPase subunit defective in an inherited form of distal renal tubular acidosis. *J Am Soc Nephrol*, *14*, 3027-3038.

[26] Sobacchi, C., Frattini, A., Orchard, P., Porras, O., Tezcan, I., et al. (2001). The mutational spectrum of human malignant autosomal recessive osteopetrosis. *Hum Mol Genet*, *10*, 1767-1773.

[27] Sly, W. S., Hewett-Emmett, D., Whyte, M. P., Yu, Y. S. & Tashian, R. E. (1983). Carbonic anhydrase II deficiency identified as the primary defect in the autosomal recessive syndrome of osteopetrosis with renal tubular acidosis and cerebral calcification. *Proc Natl Acad Sci U S A*, *80*, 2752-2756.

[28] Lima, F. B., Ota, F. H., Cabral, F. J., Del Bianco Borges, B. & Franci, C. R. (2014). Estrogen, but not progesterone, induces the activity of nitric oxide synthase within the medial preoptic area in female rats. *Brain research*, *1578*, 23-29.

[29] Sorkin, A. & von Zastrow, M. (2009). Endocytosis and signalling: intertwining molecular networks. *Nat Rev Mol Cell Biol*, *10*, 609-622.

[30] Doherty, G. J. & McMahon, H. T. (2009). Mechanisms of endocytosis. *Annu Rev Biochem*, *78*, 857-902.

[31] Recchi, C. & Chavrier, P. (2006). V-ATPase: a potential pH sensor. *Nat Cell Biol*, *8*, 107-109.

[32] Mindell, J. A. (2012). Lysosomal acidification mechanisms. *Annu Rev Physiol*, *74*, 69-86.

[33] Arnold, K., Bordoli, L., Kopp, J. & Schwede, T. (2006). The SWISS-MODEL workspace: a web-based environment for protein structure homology modelling. *Bioinformatics*, *22*, 195-201.

In: Handbook of Hearing Disorders Research
Editor: Charlotte Hailee Atkinson

ISBN: 978-1-63463-654-4

Chapter 7

Novel Deafness Genes and Mutations Identified by Next Generation Sequencing

Xue Gao[1,2,*]
[1]Department of Otorhinolaryngology, Head and Neck Surgery, PLA General Hospital, Beijing, Haidian, China
[2]Department of Otolaryngology, the Second Artillery; General Hospital, Beiging, China

Abstract

Identifying the genetic basis of deafness provides crucial information for diagnosis, intervention and treatment of the disease. Non-syndromic sensorineural hearing loss, however, are extremely heterogeneous, with both common and rare forms occurring due to mutations over estimated 500 genes. Due to the larger number and presumably low mutation frequencies of those genes, it would be highly expensive and time-consuming to address this issue by conventioanl gene-by-gene Sanger sequencing. Next generation sequencing (NGS) has become a highly efficient strategy for identifying novel causative genes and mutations involved in heritable disease. Both simple nonsyndromic and complex syndromic forms of hearing loss can be resolved efficiently using NGS, especially in small families with distinct and interesting phenotypes that were once too small to map. To date, more than a dozen syndromic or nonsyndromic deafness genes have been identified using targeted genomic enrichment and NGS. Here, we summarized novel deafness genes and mutations identified by NGS methodologies.

Introduction

To date, more than 100 genes and 100 genetic loci have been implicated in NSHL (http://hereditaryhearingloss.org/). The marked heterogeneity of genetic hearing loss can be

* Corresponding author: Xue Gao. E-mail: mixueer0110@126.com.

explained by the complexity of the auditory system, which requires coordination of multiple processes involving the inner ear and nervous system. A defect in any part of this complex chain of events can lead to hearing impairment. For many decades, linkage analysis has been the most powerful and widely used strategy to identify the gene defects responsible for inherited disorders. However, this approach is time consuming and requires the availability of cohorts of homogeneous and informative, possibly large families and a large proportion of NSHL remain genetically unexplained.

These limitations, however, may be overcome by the next-generation sequencing (NGS) technologies. NGS offers an unprecedented ability to identify rare variants and new causative genes. Several next generation sequencing platforms allow for a DNA-to-diagnosis protocol to identify the molecular basis of inherited non-syndromic hearing loss, including whole genome sequencing (WGS), whole exome sequencing (WES) and targeted deafness gene capture. Updated guidelines from the American College of Medical Genetics and Genomics (ACMG) recommend that clinicians consider NGS when testing for genetic causes of hearing loss [1]. The guideline, which is build on guidelines issued in 2002, include panel tests targeted at genes related to hearing loss, whole exome sequencing, and whole genome sequencing after negative results are returned on initial single-gene testing indicated by a patient's family medical history and presentation.

Whole Genome Sequencing

Whole genome sequencing (WGS) by next generation sequencing technologies has the potential for simultaneous, comprehensive, differential diagnostic testing of monogenic illnesses.

In 2003, the cost of sequencing a single human genome was estimated to be 2.7 billion dollars, that price had dropped to 4,000 dollars by 2012, and it is anticipated that this cost will soon be 1,000 dollars. Clinical use of WGS by NGS has taken at least a month. Researchers already have been able to help clinicians aid some children born with rare birth defects by sequencing and analyzing their whole genomes to diagnose and treat their illness [2].

This is only the beginning of the whole genome sequencing era, which has the potential to revolutionize medicine.

However, there is no report about application of whole genome seuqencing on the inherited non-syndromic hearing loss. There are major obstacles to the clinical implementation of WGS, such as hidden costs, issues surrounding sequencing and analysis, quality assurance and standardization protocols, ethical dilemmas, and difficulties with interpretation of the results. With the availability of human WGS data from many individuals, it's now clear that two unrelated individuals have at least two million differences in their genomic DNA sequences [3]. The full potential of WGS can be realized only when we gain a much better understanding of the functions of noncoding regions. WGS should be carefully implemented in the clinic to allow the realization of its potential to improve patient health in specific indications.

Whole Exome Sequencing

Approximately 85% of disease-related mutations in Mendelian disorders have been found in the protein-coding region, although this portion constitutes only approximately 1% of the human genome [4, 5]. WES has become a highly efficient strategy for identifying novel causative genes and mutations involved in heritable disease.

Over 1,778 publications since 2009 whose abstracts contain the term "whole exome sequencing", confirm the success of exome sequencing as a new and effective technological paradigm within human genetics.

Whole exome sequencing has proven useful for identifyding the molecular defects underlying single gene disorders (Mendelian inheritance), as well as some genetically heterogeneous disorders, such as inherited non-syndromic hearing loss.

Inherited non-syndromic hearing loss can be resolved efficiently using WES, especially in small families with distinct and interesting phenotypes that were once too small to map using linkage analysis.

Recently, there have been many successful applications of WES in identifying the causative genes and mutations of inherited non-syndromic hearing loss (table 1).

Table 1. List of genes and mutations related with non-syndromic hearing loss identified by WES

GENE NAME	Mutation (protein)	References
OSBPL2	p.Gln53Argfs*100 p.Leu195Met	[6]
TBC1D24	p.Ser178Leu	[7]
TNC	p. Thr 1796Ser p.V1773M	[8]
ELMOD3	p.Leu265Ser	[9]
KARS	p.Asp377Asn p.Tyr173His	[10]
GRXCR2	c.714dupT	[11]
ATP1A2	p.Val191Met	[12]
ADCY1	p.Arg1038X	[13]
BDP1	p.*2625Gluext*11	[14]
EPS8	p.Gln30*	[15]
PNKP	p.Gly292Arg	[16]
PCDH15	p.Met65Ile p.Ser404Arg	[16]
CDH23	p.Pro240Leu p.Glu1595Lys p.Asn342Ser	[17]
POU4F3	p.Arg326Lys	[18]
MYO15A	p.Ser1481 Pro p.Gln1425X p.Ala1551Asp IVS11 + 1 p.Arg2146Q	[19, 20, 21]
TMC1	p.Ser530X p.Gly197Arg p.Gln391X	[19, 22]

Table 1. (Continued)

GENE NAME	Mutation (protein)	References
ACTG1	p.Met305Thr	[23]
LOXHD1	p. Arg1494X p. Glu955X	[19]
GIPC3	p.His170Asn	[19]
ILDR1	p. Gln 274X	[19]
MYO7A	p.Gly2163 Ser	[19]
TECTA	p. Tyr 1737Cys	[19]
TMPRSS3	p.F13Lfs*10	[19]
TRIOBP	p. Arg785 Ser fs*50	[19]

To date, 10 non-syndromic deafness genes and more than 30 novel causative mutations were identified by WES (Table 1). These studies show that WES, followed by verification and functional and immunolabeling examinations, can reveal critical disease-causing genes from small pedigrees.

Even with the rapid maturarion of this field, there are a number of areas that are still many work in progress: (1) WES fails to solve a substantial proportion of presumably Mendelian phenotypes [24]. (2) There is tremendous interest understanding the contribution of rare variation to the genetic basis of common disease. Many such studies have been initiated using WES, but are still ongoing as they require other samples to tesifty the results. (3) The discrete prioritazation of all protein-altering variation over all other variations has clearly proven to be useful, but is undeniably crude.

Targeted Deafness Gene Capture and NGS

The popular application of targeted gene capture is all of the genes involved in causing hearing loss, including all exons, exon/intron boundaries and promoter sequences could be fully sequenced on a diagnostic platform to produce a specific genetic test for hearing loss. Targeted deafness gene capture combined with NGS is suited to identify the causative mutations of non-syndromic hereditary hearing loss owing to the following advantages: 1) comprehensive coverage of large numbers of genes and large genes associated with the disease; 2) significant cost saving; 3) higher sequencing accuracy because of deeper achievable coverage; 4) a significantly shorter turnaround time and 5) more convincing dataset by excluding other deafness genes [25].

To date, more than 100 human genes implicated in non-syndromic hearing loss are confirmed [25]. Approximately 100Gbp of sequencing is needed to obtain NGS results for one human genome (~3.2G bp) at about 30× average coverage. Targeted gene enrichment typically increases this proportion by at least 1,000 fold [26, 27, 28].

Therefore, the same sequencing capacity can theoretically be used to sequence more than 1,000 samples for a panel of genes associated with deafness.

The recent studies demonstrated the feasibility of conducting diagnostic tests for all deafness-related genes by targeted gene capture and NGS [26, 27]. Its success in research has already resulted in its translational uses in clinical care, and many of them are for diagnostic mutation detection of focused panels of disease genes.

OtoSCOPE (Otological Sequence Capture Of Pathogenic Exons) is the first massively parallel sequencing platform that utilizes targeted sequence capture and NGS for genetic testing of hearing loss [27]. It has been developed by the University of Iowa and is being used in a research setting to fully sequence all exons of 57 deafness genes (http://www.healthcare.uiowa.edu/ labs/morl/index_CDS.htm). At this stage in its development various methods of targeted sequence capture and NGS are being compared to determine which combination has the greatest level of sequence coverage. Otogenetics Corporation in the US is currently offering a genetic mutation testing service using targeted sequence capture and NGS for the detection of variants in 131 known deafness genes for approximately $500 per sample (www.otogenetics. com). Richard J.H. Smith, MD, Director of the Molecular Otolaryngology and Renal Research Laboratories at the Iowa Institute of Human Genetics at University of Iowa in Iowa City, is a proponent of panel testing for hearing loss. His lab offers a test that covers 90 genes known to cause hearing loss, which he suggests over any initial single-gene test. Because panel tests offer more depth of coverage in genes associated with hearing loss, they are superior to WES at some extent, which looks at 20,000 genes and may miss parts of them. The drawbacks of panel tests are these tests that use disease-targeted exon capture focused on specific genes may only sequence a subset of the genes known to cause hearing loss, and there is limited knowledge of which genes are involved in hearing loss.

Challenge and Future

Applications of NGS technologies are now beginning to enter clinical practice. Interpreting the data and translating the research results into applications that improve healthcare is still challenging. Filtering through the millions of vatiants in an individual's genome for the pathogenic mutation seems to be the most urgent task at hand. Another important aspect is the concurrent development of genetic counseling capabilities to interpret the large amount of data revealed by NGS for clinical use. In the near future, physicians may combine a past medical history and family history with NGS diagnostic data to identity disease predisposition vatiants and variants that affect drug metabolism in individuals.

Althoght NGS-based molecular diagnostic tests are still in their infancy, they have demonstrated excellent clinical utility for single-gene disorders. With further developments in NGS technologies for data generation and with more effective bioinformatics tools for data analysis and clinical extraction, the full potential of WES/WGS that we expect to be revealed in the coming years will greatly enrich and empower the practice of genomic medicine beyond the rare single-gene disorders. The improvements in patient care demonstrated in recent studies justify all effort and cost for moving these new and exciting approaches into molecular diagnostics practics.

In our opinion, WES, WGS, and targeted deafness gene capture should remain as options to be considered for inherited non-syndromic hearing loss and be used according to a patient's specific conditions. Alternatively, a combined approach can be used to capture all variety of genomic variations.

References

[1] Levenson, D. (2014) New testing guidelines for hearing loss support next-generation sequencing: testing method may help determine genetic causes of hearing loss among patients whose phenotypes are not easily distinguished clinically. *Am. J. Med. Genet.* A 164: vii-viii.

[2] Saunders, C. J., Miller, N. A., Soden, S. E., Dinwiddie, D. L., Noll, A., et al. (2012) Rapid whole-genome sequencing for genetic disease diagnosis in neonatal intensive care units. *Sci. Transl. Med.* 4: 154ra135.

[3] Moore, B., Hu, H., Singleton, M., De La Vega, F. M., Reese, M. G., et al. (2011) Global analysis of disease-related DNA sequence variation in 10 healthy individuals: implications for whole genome-based clinical diagnostics. *Genet. Med.* 13: 210-217.

[4] Ng, S. B., Turner, E. H., Robertson, P. D., Flygare, S. D., Bigham, A. W., et al. (2009) Targeted capture and massively parallel sequencing of 12 human exomes. *Nature* 461: 272-276.

[5] Teer, J. K., Mullikin, J. C. (2010) Exome sequencing: the sweet spot before whole genomes. *Hum. Mol. Genet.* 19: R145-151.

[6] Xing, G., Yao, J., Wu, B., Liu, T., Wei, Q., et al. (2014) Identification of OSBPL2 as a novel candidate gene for progressive nonsyndromic hearing loss by whole-exome sequencing. *Genet. Med.*

[7] Azaiez, H., Booth, K. T., Bu, F., Huygen, P., Shibata, S. B., et al. (2014) TBC1D24 mutation causes autosomal-dominant nonsyndromic hearing loss. *Hum. Mutat.* 35: 819-823.

[8] Zhao, Y., Zhao, F., Zong, L., Zhang, P., Guan, L., et al. (2013) Exome sequencing and linkage analysis identified tenascin-C (TNC) as a novel causative gene in nonsyndromic hearing loss. *PLoS One* 8: e69549.

[9] Jaworek, T. J., Richard, E. M., Ivanova, A. A., Giese, A. P., Choo, D. I., et al. (2013) An alteration in ELMOD3, an Arl2 GTPase-activating protein, is associated with hearing impairment in humans. *PLoS Genet.* 9: e1003774.

[10] Santos-Cortez, R. L., Lee, K., Azeem, Z., Antonellis, P. J., Pollock, L. M., et al. (2013) Mutations in KARS, encoding lysyl-tRNA synthetase, cause autosomal-recessive nonsyndromic hearing impairment DFNB89. *Am. J. Hum. Genet.* 93: 132-140.

[11] Imtiaz, A., Kohrman, D. C., Naz, S. (2014) A frameshift mutation in GRXCR2 causes recessively inherited hearing loss. *Hum. Mutat.* 35: 618-624.

[12] Oh, S. K., Baek, J. I., Weigand, K. M., Venselaar, H., Swarts, H. G., et al. (2014) A missense variant of the ATP1A2 gene is associated with a novel phenotype of progressive sensorineural hearing loss associated with migraine. *Eur. J. Hum. Genet.*

[13] Santos-Cortez, R. L., Lee, K., Giese, A. P., Ansar, M., Amin-Ud-Din, M., et al. (2014) Adenylate cyclase 1 (ADCY1) mutations cause recessive hearing impairment in humans and defects in hair cell function and hearing in zebrafish. *Hum. Mol. Genet.* 23: 3289-3298.

[14] Girotto, G., Abdulhadi, K., Buniello, A., Vozzi, D., Licastro, D., et al. (2013) Linkage study and exome sequencing identify a BDP1 mutation associated with hereditary hearing loss. *PLoS One* 8: e80323.

[15] Behlouli, A., Bonnet, C., Abdi, S., Bouaita, A., Lelli, A., et al. (2014) EPS8, encoding an actin-binding protein of cochlear hair cell stereocilia, is a new causal gene for autosomal recessive profound deafness. *Orphanet J. Rare Dis.* 9: 55.

[16] Nakashima, M., Takano, K., Osaka, H., Aida, N., Tsurusaki, Y., et al. (2014) Causative novel PNKP mutations and concomitant PCDH15 mutations in a patient with microcephaly with early-onset seizures and developmental delay syndrome and hearing loss. *J. Hum. Genet.* 59: 471-474.

[17] Woo, H. M., Park, H. J., Park, M. H., Kim, B. Y., Shin, J. W., et al. (2014) Identification of CDH23 mutations in Korean families with hearing loss by whole-exome sequencing. *BMC Med. Genet.* 15: 46.

[18] Kim, H. J., Won, H. H., Park, K. J., Hong, S. H., Ki, C. S., et al. (2013) SNP linkage analysis and whole exome sequencing identify a novel POU4F3 mutation in autosomal dominant late-onset nonsyndromic hearing loss (DFNA15). *PLoS One* 8: e79063.

[19] Diaz-Horta, O., Duman, D., Foster, J., 2nd, Sirmaci, A., Gonzalez, M., et al. (2012) Whole-exome sequencing efficiently detects rare mutations in autosomal recessive nonsyndromic hearing loss. *PLoS One* 7: e50628.

[20] Gao, X., Zhu, Q. Y., Song, Y. S., Wang, G. J., Yuan, Y. Y., et al. (2013) Novel compound heterozygous mutations in the MYO15A gene in autosomal recessive hearing loss identified by whole-exome sequencing. *J. Transl. Med.* 11: 284.

[21] Woo, H. M., Park, H. J., Baek, J. I., Park, M. H., Kim, U. K., et al. (2013) Whole-exome sequencing identifies MYO15A mutations as a cause of autosomal recessive nonsyndromic hearing loss in Korean families. *BMC Med. Genet.* 14: 72.

[22] Gao, X., Su, Y., Guan, L. P., Yuan, Y. Y., Huang, S. S., et al. (2013) Novel compound heterozygous TMC1 mutations associated with autosomal recessive hearing loss in a Chinese family. *PLoS One* 8: e63026.

[23] Park, G., Gim, J., Kim, A. R., Han, K. H., Kim, H. S., et al. (2013) Multiphasic analysis of whole exome sequencing data identifies a novel mutation of ACTG1 in a nonsyndromic hearing loss family. *BMC Genomics* 14: 191.

[24] Fairfield, H., Gilbert, G. J., Barter, M., Corrigan, R. R., Curtain, M., et al. (2011) Mutation discovery in mice by whole exome sequencing. *Genome Biol.* 12: R86.

[25] Lin, X., Tang, W., Ahmad, S., Lu, J., Colby, C. C., et al. (2012) Applications of targeted gene capture and next-generation sequencing technologies in studies of human deafness and other genetic disabilities. *Hear. Res.* 288: 67-76.

[26] Brownstein, Z., Friedman, L. M., Shahin, H., Oron-Karni, V., Kol, N., et al. (2011) Targeted genomic capture and massively parallel sequencing to identify genes for hereditary hearing loss in Middle Eastern families. *Genome Biol.* 12: R89.

[27] Shearer, A. E., DeLuca, A. P., Hildebrand, M. S., Taylor, K. R., Gurrola, J., 2nd, et al. (2010) Comprehensive genetic testing for hereditary hearing loss using massively parallel sequencing. *Proc. Natl. Acad. Sci. US* 107: 21104-21109.

[28] Tang, W., Qian, D., Ahmad, S., Mattox, D., Todd, N. W., et al. (2012) A low-cost exon capture method suitable for large-scale screening of genetic deafness by the massively-parallel sequencing approach. *Genet. Test Mol. Biomarkers* 16: 536-542.

In: Handbook of Hearing Disorders Research
Editor: Charlotte Hailee Atkinson
ISBN: 978-1-63463-654-4

Chapter 8

Conduct Disorder in Children and Youth with Hearing Impairment

Fadilj Eminovic** and Sanja Dimoski
Faculty of Special Education and Rehabilitation,
University of Belgrade, Belgrade, Serbia

Abstract

Hearing impairment is a condition that involves medical, psychological and social aspects. Surveys report that children and adolescents with hearing impairment show high prevalence of psychopathology. Among numerous definitions which are largely overlapping (Oppositional Defiant Disorders, Externalizing Disorder, Behavior Problems, Socio-emotional Problems), we have chosen the definition of conduct disorder given by the World Health Organization in ICD -10. Some of the criteria for the diagnosis are: violation of the rules of adults, frequent anger and resentment, deliberate destruction of other people's property. The aim of this paper is to examine the relationships between hearing impairment and conduct disorder. The survey was conducted in Serbia, the environment characterized by specific circumstances concerning the educational and socio-economic conditions. This society has not developed a tradition of inclusive education for children, and inclusive trends are slow in general. The study was conducted on 375 patients of whom 169 are with a hearing impairment, and 178 with no hearing impairment. The respondents with hearing impairment attended school for hearing-impaired children. Some of the respondents with hearing impairment live in abroad school and some with their families. As an instrument, we used a scale for assessing behavioral disorders (Dimoski, 2004), which was filled by the specialists working in the institutions for children and youth with hearing impairments. The survey did not show statistically significant differences in the presence of behavioral disorders in the sample without hearing impairment and the sample of individuals with hearing impairment. However, the results showed that the children with hearing impairment showed significantly greater degree of two indicators of behavioral disorders - the tendency to steal ($t = -3.18$, $p = 0.002$) and extortion of money or benefit from the younger or weaker

* Corresponding author's email: eminovic73@gmail.com.

(t = -2.07, p = 0.039). This paper also deals with correlates of behavioral disorders in all patients (sex, age, academic achievement, socio-economic status) and with connection to the onset, severity of hearing impairment and type of accommodation (boarding or family) in the group of patients with hearing impairment. The male respondents (t = 3:07, p = 0.003) with lower school achievement (F = 11.219, p = 0.000) have more evident indicators of behavioral disorders. This work has important implications relating to the practice of working with children and youth with hearing impairment. It was recommended to work on prevention of behavioral disorders, and suggested which types of psychosocial interventions for those who express this disorder may be used.

Keywords: Hearing impairment, conduct disorder, children, youth, practice of working

Conduct Disorder in Children and Youth with Hearing Impairment

Problematic behavior in children and adolescents is a common subject of studies in contemporary researches. It is approached to these researches from the perspective of psychology, psychiatry, pedagogy and other related scientific fields. The research of problematic behavior in children and adolescents is followed by methodological difficulties related to the lack of precise terminology used to determine the object of study, and various criteria by which certain manifestations of behavior are treated as problematic behavior in children and adolescents. The large number of various definitions, which are often at least partially overlapping is used. The terms: antisocial behavior, externalized behavioral problems, oppositional defiant disorder, behavioral problems, socio-emotional problems, conduct disorder, and specific criteria that define this phenomenon were used. In Serbian language the terms that are in common use are: juvenile offenders and delinquents. There are also various categorical and dimensional approaches to the definition of these phenomena.

The approaches of the researchers are not in compliance neither. Some senior researchers support the attitude that antisocial behavior in childhood and adolescents is a unique syndrome, regardless of variety of symptoms relating to the phenomenon (Robins, 1966, Robins & Ratcliff, 1980) while many recent studies, as well as factor analysis do not confirm this hypothesis. Summing up the results of the factor analysis of a large number of different studies, it was concluded that the problematic behavior of children can best be conceptualized on the basis of two dimensions, namely discovered-hidden dimensions and destructive-non-destructive dimension (Frick et al., 1993).

In *Diagnostic and Statistical Manual* (DSM-IV) conduct disorder is related to the repeated and persistent patterns of behavior that violates the basic rights of others and the general norms and rules appropriate to age (aggression toward people and animals, destruction of property, deceitfulness or theft, and serious violation of rules).

In modern dimensional systems the division of the externalized and internalized behavior problems is accepted (Achenbach & Rescorla, 2001). We have isolated two externalized syndrome, which are only partially consistent with the diagnosis of DSM-IV. The first syndrome, called aggressive behavior, includes oppositional defiant behavior and aggressive conduct disorder, while other syndrome, so-called behavior that violates the rules, includes only non-aggressive forms of behavior disorders. This division implies the existence of two types of behavioral disorders. The first "discovered" or "aggressive" type, characterized by hostile confrontations with others, either in the form of a legal opposition or aggressive behavior, and other "hidden" or "non-aggressive" type includes symptoms of conduct disorder, which does not includes a confrontation with the victim, substance abuse and association with delinquent peers (Loeber & Schmaling, 1985).

We have accepted the definition of conduct disorder offered by the World Health Organization ICD-10, 1993. In the scientific and professional practice in Serbia none of the definitions is unanimously accepted. Determination of the ICD-10 is largely used in clinical work with children and young people with this kind of disorder which led us to choose this definition. Some of the criteria for the diagnosis of conduct disorder are: often reluctance or refusal of requests and rules of adults, deliberately destroying other people's property, sensitivity and tendency to be annoyed by others (*Often touchy or easily annoyed by others*), frequent anger and resentment (*Often angry or resentful*) excessive fighting with other children, excluding children in the family (*Excessive fighting with other children, with frequent initiation of fights (not including fights with siblings*), criminogenic episodes involving confrontation with the victim - intimidation, extortion, frequent truancy from school beginning before 13 years of age. It is considered that it is more significant for the foresight to take into account the severity and not the exact type of symptoms. During diagnosis, manifestations of behavioral disorders that last no less than six months and are not isolated antisocial acts are taken into account. This classification makes a distinction between socialized, none-socialized and oppositional defiant disorder.

The existence of different approaches in diagnosing the problematic behavior in childhood is a major reason for the inconsistency of the data on their prevalence. In a study in which the criteria of the DSM are applied, the prevalence of conduct disorder among children and adolescents ranges from 1% to 9%, while the opposition defiant disorder is not so present, with prevalence of about 2% (Essau, 2003). Frequency of externalized problems in the total population of children and adolescents ranges between 2% and 15% (Hinshaw, 1992). Conduct disorder, which involves persistent patterns of rule-breaking and violent behavior, is estimated to have a prevalence of 9% for boys and 2% for girls (Offord et al, 1986). In Serbia, the research Zunic-Pavlovic et al, (2009) shows that 12% of students exhibited antisocial behavior, and in 6% of the deficit of social competence and antisocial behavior is present.

The presence of psychopathology during developmental period in children and adolescents with hearing impairment is a frequent subject of study. Also, the presence of behavioral problems of children and youth with hearing impairments has been studied, although in this area there are several approaches of the authors and defining disorder. However, the development of research dealing with the presence of specific behavioral disorders in children and adolescents in this population is absent.

Imprecise terminology and a variety of criteria for diagnosis are followed by specific methodological difficulties related to the procedures and instruments by which we determine the presence of problem behavior in children and young people with hearing impairment. Assessment of children is difficult, due to the inability of deaf children to understand verbal instructions or verbal tasks placed before them, and the limited expressive aspects of language and speech. Experts generally do not have enough experience or social skills to conduct diagnostic assessments and are not familiar with sign language. Sometimes they include sign language interpreters, whose presence necessarily affects the tested situation. The presence of behavioral disorders is generally assessed based on the reports of parents and teachers, and some research suggests peer evaluation about the functioning of a particular child in the school context. However, estimates of the parents must not be objective, and are often saturated by subjective interpretations of children's behavior. Some authors (Van Gent, 2007) believe that the most reliable are the estimates of experts. In addition, certain symptoms (especially those related to internalized problems) have distinct subjective tone and are best detected on the basis of introspection.

In Serbia, the studying of children and youth with impaired hearing by psychologically measuring instruments is accompanied by the difficulties related to the lack of a standardized sign language in which it would be possible to translate the items of the instrument, as well as a shortage of professionals who are trained in the diagnosis of psychopathology, developmental age of this specific population. Families and children and youth with hearing impairments use the expression of spontaneous gestural communication to achieve communication. Schools and medical facilities for persons with impaired hearing have no systematized praxis on the field of communication using the sign language.

Contemporary research practice is followed by attitude that different variables, which are often not sufficiently controlled in research studies of personality of children and youth with hearing impairments (speech development, the degree of experiential, emotional, social and educational deprivation, etiology and time of occurrence of hearing loss, the time of initiation and duration of rehabilitation, the existence of cochlear implants, etc.) strongly influence the results of this group of people on personality tests. This situation is particularly applicable to the assessment of the developmental period of psychopathology, including the presence of a behavioral disorder. In studies dealing with psychopathology developmental age of children and youth with hearing loss in our society, the control of the relevant variables often lack. This particularly concerns the variables related to socio-emotional deprivation of children and youth with hearing impairments characteristics of dynamics of family relationships and the conditions of education and rehabilitation.

In Serbia, the children and young people with hearing impairment attend almost exclusively special schools for education of this population and a large number of them is housed in dormitories, or are separated from their families, already at the preschool level. A significant percentage of children and youth with hearing impairments who are educated in this system of special education have not enough well-developed language and speech abilities. The percentage of children with cochlear implants is negligible.

The importance of language and verbal abilities for adequate development many studies have emphasized. Quirin & Lane (2012) show that poor language skills can cause difficulties in understanding the social environment and, in turn, are related to an impaired emotion understanding. Many studies suggest that a delay in language development of children and youth with hearing impairment is in connection with serious difficulties in developing a proper understanding of emotion (Rieff & Terwogt 2006; Meerum Terwogt & Rieff, 2004). Some studies (Dammayer, 2009) even show that good oral or sign communication with the environment is in relation to the normal prevalence of psychosocial problems in deaf children and youth.

These difficulties may explain that the prevalence rates of mental disorders in hearing-impaired children and adolescents found in the literature vary from 15% to 60% (Bailly et al., 2003). Some studies provide disturbing data on the prevalence of psychiatric disorders in young people with hearing impairment. Hindly (1994) provides information about more than

50% of children between 11 and 16 years, Colvin et al. (1979) cites 54%. Van Gent et al, (2007) provide a comprehensive overview of recent studies of psychopathology in children and adolescents with hearing impairment analysis instruments for the evaluation. Their research indicates elevated levels of psychopathology. However, some studies do not confirm a difference in the manifestation of symptoms of psychopathology in a population of deaf and hearing respondents. Sinnkoen (1994) confirmed the slightly higher incidence of psychopathology in young people with hearing impairment, but this difference was not statistically significant.

Hearing impairment among children affects psychosocial development, but there is no consensus about the rate of prevalence. Older studies (Meadow, 1980, Freeman et al., 1975) suggest prevalence of 8-23% presence of socio-emotional problems. The largest number of recent studies (Vostanis et al., 1997; van Eldik, 1994; van Eldik et al, 2004) confirms these results. Dammajer (2009) states that studies that were performed in the last two decades provide data on the prevalence of psychosocial problems in childhood from 20% to 50%. However, the findings of the authors from Belgium, Maes & Grietens (2004) did not find elevated levels of these disorders in deaf children that were assessed by parents. Bailly et al. (2003) reported that some studies have shown the presence of normal levels of behavior emotional functioning of deaf children and youth.

Older studies (Schlesinger & Meadow, 1971), which gave information about the elevated levels of behavioral problems in this population, were the impetus for further research. Children with hearing loss have a higher level of externalized behavioral problems (30-38% van Eldik; Vostanis, et al., 1997) than children with normal hearing. Mitchell & Quittner (1996) reported that half or one-third of children and adolescents with hearing impairment (depending on whether they are evaluated by parents or teachers) exhibit behavior problems. Regarding behavioral disorder studies indicate the presence of a 12% and 14% of children and adolescents with hearing impairment compared to 7% in the control group (Hintermair, 2007). Expert's estimates show the presence of behavioral disorders in 11% of children and youth with hearing impairments (Van Gent, 2007).

Complex relations between neurological, family and social factors are basis of conduct disorders in children and adolescents with hearing impairment (Meadow, 1980). Theoretical perspectives on this issue are related to assumptions about the specific environmental conditions of children with hearing impairments which affect their emotional development or lead to the manifestation of behavioral problems. Family environment, in this respect, has a very important role. Difficulty in verbal communication and gestures between parents and hearing impaired children strongly influence the overall development of children, not just the transfer of information. Conditions of wider social environment are related to environmental factors, the socio-economic, through general social factors, conditions, rehabilitation and education, and especially terms of social acceptance of people with hearing impairment, contributes to the development or maintenance of various psychopathological symptoms.

Attempts to understand the development of conduct disorder in contemporary literature range from taking into account the role of genetic and biological predisposition over the characteristics of temperament, socio-cultural context, family relationships, experience rejection by peers, social-cognitive factors etc.

Contemporary concepts are characterized by eclectic approach to the authors and involve the effects of multiple factors in the development of the disorder and emphasize the need for verification of theoretical concepts in empirical research. Many models are a synthesis of different theoretical approaches and research findings (Moffitt, 1993; Patterson & Yoerger, 1997; Lahey & Waldman, 2002, Dodge and Pettit, 2003; Frick and Morris, 2004). Dodge & Pettit (2003) offered a bio-psychosocial model of the development of chronic conduct problems. This model posits that biological dispositions and sociocultural contexts place certain children at risk in early life but that life experiences with parents, peers, and social institutions increment and mediate this risk. They point out that certain types of mutual influences that occur between predispositions, context and life experiences of the child or adolescent, may contribute to the occurrence of behavioral disorders. In the process of developing this disorder cognitive and emotional processes play the role of mediator.

The nature of conduct disorders, as defined by ICD-10 criteria is related to the expression of resistance and aggressiveness towards the environment (peers, adults, things, institutions, rules, etc.). We believe that we should take into account the hypothesis on the tendency of children and youth with hearing loss to a more distinct expression of aggression through such nonverbal (behavioral) ways, rather than through verbal, which are not sufficiently developed for this population. The expression of emotions, including aggression in children and adolescents with hearing impairment is different than the normal hearing children and youth. As stated Rieff et al. (2003) recent findings have shown that deaf children have a different rationale for the emergence of emotions than their hearing peers. They have restricted opportunities to learn from their own and others' experiences in this respect. The research of Reiff & Terwogt (2006) showed that deaf children employed the communicative function of anger expression differently from hearing children. Whereas hearing children used anger expression to reflect on the anguish that another child caused them, deaf children used it rather bluntly and explained less.

One of the few epidemiological studies of the presence of psychopathology in children and youth impaired in our community (Tadić, 1998) dealt with the presence of behavioral problems. This study demonstrated the presence of lying in 3.2% of subjects with impaired hearing, conflicts with friends in 8% of patients, conflicts with teachers at 3.2%, and the fits of rage, breaking objects and hitting the 8.8% of respondents.

Research are trying to detect variables that may be associated with conduct disorders - gender, age, academic achievement, socio-emotional status, the nature of relationships with peers, especially the experience of rejection by peers, characteristics of temperament, character relationships with parents, the influence of parental styles of parents, presence of criminal and maladjustment behavior in close environment... When it comes to children and youth with hearing impairments in personality tests of the population, usually controlled variables affecting the degree of hearing loss are the occurrence of the hearing loss, rehabilitation characteristics, ways of communication with the environment and especially in the family and etc. We will discuss the variables in more details that are often taken into account in the various studies, which are included in this research.

Surveys consistently show a statistically significant relation between conduct disorder and half of respondents. Boys are more prone to these impairments than girls (Friedrich et al. 1984; Kerr et al. 2004; Björkqvist et al. 1992; Cohen et al. 1993; Crick, 1995; Grotpeter & Crick, 1995; Feehan et al., 1994; Offord et al. 1987, Keenan & Loeber, 1994). Peterson (1961) showed that age comparison showed that boys displayed more severe conduct problems than girls at all age levels. From about 4 years of age, boys are more likely than girls to engage in conduct problems (Keenan & Shaw, 1997; Moffitt et al., 2001; Lahey et al., 2000, Tremblay et al., 1996). Lahey et al. (2000) find that the behavioral problems of youth can not be explained without taking into account the gender (and age) differences. These authors, in a large sample of respondents aged 9 to 17 years found that boys were more likely to express aggression, and to have a common property, and misdemeanor offenses. Instead of physical aggression, females tend to use indirect, verbal and relational aggression. Moffit et al. (2001) present new findings on a number of subjects of both sexes from 3 to 21 years aligning approaches of developmental psychology, psychiatry and criminology. They suggest the need for revision of the diagnostic criteria of conduct disorder suitable for girls. Study Keenan et al. (1999) report on studies of behavioral disorders limitation only regarding boys. They believe that understanding gender differences in the course and severity of conduct disorder may lead to important information about etiology.

Research findings on the relation of conduct disorders and academic achievement are consistent, and an interest in author large. Children and adolescents of lower academic achievement are more likely to express behavioral disorder than those of academic achievement. Antisocial behavior is treated as a variable that has a negative impact on academic achievement throughout the years of educating (Bardone et al., 1996; Stott, 1981, Hawkins et al., 2003, Masten et al., 1995; Williams & McGee, 1994). Research (Dodge & Pettit, 2003; Hinshaw, 1992; Maguin & Loeber, 1996; Hinshaw & Anderson, 1996) show that externalized behavioral problems (externalizing behavior) are quite stable in early childhood, the relationship between antisocial behavior and academic skills may establish more in pre-school period and in the later period, this relationship becomes more apparent.

The researchers' interest was stimulated by the fact that the existence of behavioral problems of children with poor school achievement represents an impairment which required professional intervention. But the presence of lower academic achievement phenomenon can not be seen only in the educational context, since it can lead to self-esteem deficits and interpersonal difficulties (Mann & Brady, 1988; Lagreca & Stone, 1990).

Also, the common occurrence of behavioral disorders and poor academic achievement may be treated as a clear predictor of later lack of adaptation in adolescence, which can lead to antisocial behavior and substance abuse (Hinshaw, 1992). Vostanis et al. (1997) found that poor functioning in school variable best predicts the presence of behavioral and emotional problems in children and adolescents with hearing impairment. Many authors (Williams & McGree, 1994) pointed out the importance of reading skills in commonly injured children and youth with hearing impairments and their relationship with challenging behavior.

Developed research practice concerns the attempts to determine the relationships between risk factors of the environment and the occurrence of antisocial behavior. Environmental effects, those related to family and related to the environment, highly correlate (Ingoldsby & Shaw, 2002; Leventhal & Brooks-Gunn, 2000), although it is considered useful to separate them for a deeper understanding of the etiology (Schonberg & Shaw, 2007). From about five to six years of age, differences in conduct problems in children living in disadvantaged neighborhoods become more pronounced even after controlling family demographic characteristics (Brooks-Gunn, Duncan, Klebanov & Sealand, 1993; Chase-Landsdale & Gordon, 1996). Research findings (Lahey et al., 1999, Sampson et al., 1997), generally suggest that children and adolescents from families of lower socioeconomic status are more likely to express behavioral disorder than those from the upper. Keenan et al. (1997) have given the finding that child from low-income families in nearly 5% of express behavior disorder. Research (Hausman & Hammen, 1993; Carr, 1999) indicates the relationship of low socio-economic status, poverty and social isolation and behavioral disorders. Duncan et al.

(1994) find that it seems that the longer the child has been living in poverty within the first four years of life, the more prevalent externalizing behavior problems become.

Many studies confirm that the prevalence of conduct disorder and delinquency is in relation to the different characteristics of the immediate environment (neighborhood), including socioeconomic and cultural conditions of the general (Bursik & Grasmick, 1993; Loeber & Wikstrom, 1993, Sampson & Groves, 1989; Stouthamer- Loeber et al. 1999; Wikstrom, 1991, 1998).

Significant research data (Moffitt et al., 1996; Nagin & Tremblay, 1999) show that nearly half of all children who engage in high levels of conduct problems show considerable improvement by early adolescence. Research suggests that risk factors have a different impact on the occurrence of behavioral disturbances during development and highlights the importance of understanding these complex interactions.

Method

Participants

The total sample of this study is N = 347 respondents. Part of the sample consists of children and young people with hearing impairment (N = 169), or 48.7% of the respondents. They are students of only two special schools for pupils with hearing impairment in Belgrade, capital of Serbia. In these schools the highest percentage of children with hearing impairment are being educated, because in inclusive programs, which are defined by law only in 2013, only small percentage of children and youth is included. The sample did not include the children and young people with hearing impairment who still have some kind of associated disturbances. Regarding the degree of hearing loss, the sample consisted of (N = 120) deaf patients, or 71% of the sample (N = 49) partially deaf, hard of hearing respondents, or 29% of the sample. Hearing loss is caused by perilingualy N = 141, or 83% of the sample, a lingual with N = 28 respondents, or 17% of the sample.

Children and youth with hearing impairment attending special schools and living in the dorms, N = 107, or 63% of the sample. These are respondents whose families do not live in the Serbian capital (or other cities where there are schools for children and the youth impaired). These children leave the family in the pre-school period and the entire education live in boarding schools. The second part of the sample of children and youth impaired respondents, N = 62 who live with their families, the capital of Serbia and attend a special school for the deaf, or 37% of the sample.

The children and youth who were included in the study aged from 7 to 18 years. Included are children of eight years of primary school, and youth first three years of high school. Sample respondents with hearing loss male consisted of N = 102 and female N= 67.

As an indicator of academic achievement the sample of achievement in school subjects in the previous academic year was taken into account. This variable was divided into three categories: good or underachievement success in school, very good grades in school and excellent school. Success in school subjects with impaired hearing is the largest in the category of great success, 54% of respondents.

Considering the economy, the situation in Serbia and the transition through which the country is going, there are simple difficulties in identifying indicators of socio-economic status of the family, which would be relevant for research purposes. We have opted for the educational attainment of the respondent's father, which is one indicator of the socio-economical position of the family that often accompanies the research in our community.

This variable is divided into four categories: elementary school, finished vocational training school, high school and university or university degree. Educational level of the father is in nearly 30% of the sample primary school, or the lowest category of education in Serbia, which implies a low socio-economic position.

The control group consisted of children and young people with a normal hearing (N = 178), or 51.3% of the total sample. They are regular students of primary and secondary school in Belgrade. The sample consisted of male respondents N = 84, a female N = 94. According to school success they were distributed relatively equally in all three categories. Academic success of finished high school of the father of the respondent's is most frequent followed by fathers with secondary education, that is 40% of the sample with proper hearing.

Statistical comparison of groups of patients (with and without hearing loss) showed the following:

Group 1 was significantly different from the variable gender ($\chi2$ = 6.041, p = 0.005, Cramer's V = 0.132)

Groups are significantly different in relation to school success, subjects with impaired hearing have better academic success than subjects without hearing impairment ($\chi2$ = 15.760, p = 0.001, Cramer's V = 0.213). Explanation of this difference can be found in a weaker assessment criteria in a special school for deaf students;

Groups are significantly different compared to graduates father of respondents ($\chi2$ = 67,132, p = 0.001, Cramer's V = 0.441); Respondents with impaired hearing come from lower socioeconomic families compared with patients with normal hearing.

Instrument

In Serbia not one instrument to measure conduct disorders was used in the research practice which is used in Anglo-Saxon scientific research. Also, there are no standardized instruments that are designed for subjects with impaired hearing in this region. Therefore, we decided to use the instrument of the local authors (Dimoski, 2001), *Scale for assessment of the presence of behavioral disorders*. This instrument is filled by teachers of children and youth, the survey respondents. Assessment of teachers matched the plan of this research, given that a large percentage of respondents with impaired hearing lived away from their families, and parents often do not have the relevant data on the investigated phenomena. Some authors (Van Gent, 2007) suggest that the most reliable are the estimates of experts.

The instrument consists of 15 statements that are evaluated on a scale in which 1 point denoted the absence of manifestations of behavior disorder, 2 points, the presence of low intensity, medium presence of 3 points, 4 points expressed presence. The claims set in the instrument are mainly related to the manifestation of conduct disorder as defined in this disorder ICD-10. The instrument is accompanied by a recommendation from the ICD-10, which suggests that the manifestation of behavioral disorders should be present in the last six months.

Detailed instruction is preceded by the instrument.

Reliability of the instrument, measured by Cronbach's Alpha is 0.921. The reliability of the instrument for sample hearing impaired subjects was 0.934, and the sample of respondents without hearing damage is 0.917.

Procedure

After the detailed planning of the sample, we have started the research. The subjects with hearing impairment were evaluated by their teachers in special schools. Teachers are professionals for hearing impairments (special educators) who are well familiar with the children, at least several years. They are also their homeroom teachers or principal professional persons for training and general care of a particular child.

Subjects without hearing impairment were assessed by their teachers, homeroom teachers in regular education system.

All participants in the study who gave their assessment by filling the Scale of the the presence of conduct disorder were given detailed oral and written instructions. The purpose of the study was explained and their consent to use the results for research purposes was obtained. Previously, the consent of parents of children and youth, and school management was obtained.

Results

The main results of this study concern the estimation of the presence of conduct disorders in hearing impaired children and young people in Serbia.

Table 1. Total score on a scale of conduct disorders in a sample with and without hearing loss

Group	N	AS	SD	T	df	p
No damage	178	21.51	7.02			
With hearing damage	169	20.59	5.24	1.304	262.836	0.193

When used a total score on a scale of conduct disorders it is not possible to determine a statistically significant difference ($p = 0.193$) between patients with and without hearing impairments.

We have accessed to the additional analysis of the items of the instrument in order to supplement the basic findings of research that is not indicating the difference between the two groups in terms of the presence of conduct disorders. For the purpose of the work we have selected items which have statistically significant difference present.

The research included the identification of correlates of conduct disorders in children and adolescents with hearing impairment. The following are findings that are related to assumed variables that are related to behavioral disorders in children and adolescents with hearing impairment.

Table 2. T test for items found to have statistically significant differences in the manifestations of conduct disorders in the groups with and without damage

Item	Group	AS	SD	T	df	p
Prone to theft	No damage	1.03	0.15	3.176	208.20	0.002
	With hearing damage	1.53	0.42			
Extort money from younger or weaker students	Without damage	1.02	0.18	2.074	240.55	0.005
	With hearing damage	1.39	0.38			

Table 3. Summary scores of conduct disorder distributed according to the degree of hearing loss

Degree of hearing impairment	N	AS	SD	T	df	P
Deaf	120	19.63	4.50	-1.518	167	0.131
Hard of hearing	49	20.98	5.48			

Analysis of the total score of conduct disorder shows that in a sample of individuals with hearing loss there were no statistically significant differences ($p = 0.131$) between the deaf and hard of hearing patients. The level of impairment is not related to the presence of conduct disorders in hearing impaired children and youth.

Table 4. Total score of conduct disorders distributed by time of origin of hearing loss

Time of occurence of the hearing impairment	N	AS	SD	T	df	p
Prelingnual	141	20.67	5.10	0.449	167	0.654
Postlingual	28	20.18	5.59			

The analysis of the total scores of conduct disorder shows that in a sample of individuals with hearing loss there was no statistically significant difference ($p = 0.654$) between patients who had hearing loss caused prelingually and postlingually. Time of occurrence of the hearing impairment was not related to the presence of conduct disorders in hearing impaired children and youth.

Analysis of the total scores of conduct disorder in relation to gender shows that there is a statistically significant difference ($p = 0.003$) in the expression of conduct disorders among boys and girls with hearing impairment. Male respondents expressed a greater presence of behavioral disorders.

Table 5. Total score of conduct disorders in boys and girls with hearing impairment

Gender	N	AS	SD	t	df	p
Male	102	21.55	5.127			
Female	67	19.12	4.86	3.072	149	0.003

Table 6. T test for items in which we found statistically significant difference in the manifestations of conduct disorders in boys and girls with hearing impairment

Item	Gender	AS	SD	T	df	p
Prone to physical cruelty toward younger and weaker students	Boys	1.73	0.80			
	Girls	1.37	0.55	3.408	166	0.001
Prone to purposefully annoy others	Boys	1.75	0.78			
	Girls	1.33	0.59	3.954	164	0.000
Tends to threaten, intimidate and harass other	Boys	1.29	0.48			
	Girls	1.09	0.45	2.811	147	0.006
Prone to fights	Boysi	1.50	0.66			
	Girls	1.12	0.48	4.359	165	0.000
Destructive towards common things (eg. School inventory)	Boys	1.26	0.45			
	Girls	1.06	0.24	3.457	160	0.001

Table 7. Total score of conduct disorder scores assigned to the school success of children and youth with impaired hearing

Academic achievement	N	AS	SD
Weaker and average grades in school	32	23.34	5.59
Very good grades in school	45	21.87	6.24
Excellent grades in school	92	19.00	5.24

Table 8. Analysis of variance for scores on a scale of conduct disorders in general assigned to the school success

	The sum of squares	df	Average square	F	p
Between groups	548.587	2	274.294	11.219	0.000
Within groups	4058.419	166	24.448		
Total	4607.006	168			

Analysis of variance showed a statistically significant difference between the cumulative score on a scale of conduct disorders among respondents with hearing impairments in relation to school success (p = 0.000). Respondents with lower school achievement are more likely to express conduct disorder than those with better school achievement. Given the established statistical significance of difference between the better and worse hearing impaired students, the T test for items in which statistically significant difference was found.

Table 9. T test for items found in which a statistically significant difference in the manifestations of conduct disorders among groups with different academic success was found

Item	The sum of squares		df	The average of squares	F	p
Prone to physical cruelty toward younger and weaker students	Between groups	6.738	2	3.369	6.798	
	Within groups	82.268	166	0.496		
	Total	89.006	168			0.001
Prone to purposefully annoy others	Between groups	4.294	2	2.147	4.102	
	Within groups	86.877	166	0.523		
	Total	91.172	168			0.018
Tends to threaten, intimidate and harass other	Between groups	1.187	2	0.933	4.249	
	Within groups	36.465	166	0.220		
	Total	38.331	168			0.016
Prone to fight	Between groups	2.744	2	1.372	3.694	
	Within groups	61.658	166	0.371		
	Total	64.402	168			0.027
Destructive towards common things (eg. School inventory)	Between groups	1,314	2	0.657	4.414	
	Within groups	24.710	166	0.149		
	Total	26.024	168			0.014
Destructive towardsother persons`s things	Between groups	2.202	2	0.101	3.991	
	Within groups	45.798	166	0.276		0.020
	Total	48.000	168			
Prone to theft	Between groups	1.923	2	0.961	5.865	
	Within groups	27.213	166	0.164		
	Total	29.136	168			0.003
Prone to lying from personal reasons	Between groups	7.657	2	3.829	10.489	
	Within groups	60.591	166	0.365		
	Total	68.249	168			0.000
Unexcused absence from school	Between groups	6.974	2	3.487	9.628	
	Within groups	60.126	166	0.362		
	Total	67.101	168			0.000
Tantrums	Between groups	4.797	2	2.389	7.212	
	Within groups	55.203	166	0.333		0.001
	Total	60.000	168			
Often opposition and strife in relationships with adults	Between groups	3.109	2	1.554	4.308	
	Within groups	59.897	166	0.361		
	Total	63.003	168			0.015

Analysis of the total scores of conduct disorder in the scale shows no statistically significant difference (p = 0.341) between patients who live with their families and those living in a boarding school for children and youth impaired in relation to the presence of conduct disorders.

Table 10. Total scores of conduct disorder assigned to the residence of children and youth with hearing impairments

Residence	N	AS	SD	t	df	P
Family	107	20.88	5.67	0.954	167	0.341
Boarding school	62	20.08	4.40			

Table 11. Total scores of conduct disorder assigned to age of the respondents

Age	N	AS	SD
7-10	45	19.82	4.30
11-14	67	20.97	5.43
15-18	57	20.74	5.69

Table 12. Analysis of variance for the total score of conduct disorder scores assigned by age of the subjects with hearing impairment

	The sum of squares	df	The average of squares	F
Between groups	37.435	2	18.718	0.680
Within groups	4569.571	166	27.528	
Total	4607.006	168		

Table 13. Total score of conduct disorders distributed by educational level of the father of respondents

Educational level of father	N	AS	SD
Primary School	50	21.40	5.62
Trade school	47	21.43	5.77
High school	62	19.82	4.59
Higher or university degree	10	17.30	1.77

The results show that there is no statistically significant difference ($p = 0.508$) in the total score of conduct disorders among subjects with impaired hearing of different age.

The table shows that there is no normal distribution of the variable of educational level of the father of the hearing impaired subjects. Fathers of children and youth with hearing impairments with college or university education comprise just over 6% of this part of the sample.

Table 14. Analysis of variance for scores on a scale of conduct disorders in general distributed by educational level of father of respondents

	The sum of squares	df	The average of squares	F	p
Between groups	210.368	2	70.123	2.632	0.050
Within groups	4396.638	166	26.646		
Total	4607.006	168			

Analysis of variance showed that the differences in the educational attainment of fathers of those with hearing loss is at the limit of statistical significance (p = 0.050). Children and young people with hearing impairment from lower educational and socio-economic conditions are somewhat more likely to express conduct disorder.

Table 15. T test for the item in which was a statistically significant difference was found in the manifestations of conduct disorders in patients whose fathers have different educational level

Item	The sum of squares		df	The average of squares	F	p
Prone to lie for personal gain	Between gropus	3.507	3	1.169	2.979	
	Within groups	64.741	165	0.392		
	Total	68.249	168			0.033

Discussion

Results of this study show that children and adolescents with impaired hearing are not more prone to conduct disorder than children and youth with no impairments as indicated by the total score on a scale that measured the presence of conduct disorder (Table 1). However, analysis of the individual items of the instrument shows that children and youth with hearing impairments showed statistically more emphasized some manifestations of conduct disorders (Table 2). It is the tendency of theft and extortion of money or benefits from younger or weaker students.

The findings of our study are not in accordance with the highest number of surveys that provide information that in children and youth with hearing impairments the problematic behavior is more present, no matter how they are defined, such as: behavioral problems, antisocial behavior, externalized problems, etc. Conduct disorder, as defined by ICD-10 refers, for its quality and intensity of the serious developmental problems and in this fact should be sought the explanation of our findings. Namely, the used definitions indicate more severe developmental problems than those tested in alleged researches (Schlesinger & Meadow, 1971 Freeman, et al., 1975; Meadow, 1980; van Eldik et al., 2004; Vostanis, at al., 1997). Studying developmental problems and psychopathology in children and adolescents with hearing impairments, the authors did not specifically directed their attention to the conduct disorder, as was the case with this research. Authors Prinstein & La Greca (2004) argue that the results of the study depend on how the phenomenon that is being studied is defined (ie, delinquency, aggression, illegal offenses, and nonspecific outcomes).

On the other hand, the results on variables that are assumed to be related to conduct disorders in hearing impaired in children and young people are in accordance with the findings and theoretical assumptions about the development of conduct disorder.

Our findings indicate that conduct disorder in children and adolescents with hearing impairments, in relation to the gender of the respondents - male respondents expressed a greater tendency to disorder behaviors than female respondents. Published studies (Peterson, 1961; Friedrich et al., 1984, Kerr et al. 2004; Björkqvist et al., 1992, Cohen et al. 1993; Crick, 1995; Grotpeter & Crick, 1995; Feehan et al. 1994; Offord et al., 1987, Lahey et al., 2000,

Loeber & Keenan, 1994;) on gender differences in the presence of behavioral disorders, are consistent with our results.

In addition, the findings of our studies are consistent with the findings (Bardone et al. 1996; Stott, 1981; Hawkins et al., 2003, Masten, et al., 1995, Williams & McGee, 1994; Dodge & Pettit, 2003; Hinshaw, 1992; Maguin & Loeber, 1996; Hinshaw & Anderson, 1996) that show that children and youth of lower academic achievement are more likely to express behavioral disorder.

The results of our research show that children and young people with hearing impairment who come from lower socio-economic status, if it is used as an indicator of educational level of their fathers are more prone to disorder behaviors than those from higher status families. Our findings are consistent with studies (Lahey et al., 1999, Sampson et al., 1997) on expressed emergence of behavioral disorders in families of lower socio-economic position.

The assumptions that the variables (degree of hearing loss, the time of occurrence of hearing loss and accommodation during training - a boarding school or family) are related to conduct disorders in hearing impaired children and youth are not confirmed. Also, the age of subjects is not related to the presence of behavioral disorders in children and adolescents with hearing impairment.

The value of the findings of this study is that they suggest that in the development of conduct disorders in children and adolescents with hearing impairment the specific patterns that are related specifically to the loss of auditory communication channels are not needed. The presence of the conduct disorder is more pronounced in boys, children and adolescents of lower school achievement and those from families of lower socioeconomic status. It seems that the presence of conduct disorders in childhood and adolescence is not characteristic for children and youth with hearing impairment, that is in conjunction with the hearing loss.

On the other hand, it should be considered that the diagnosis the disorder involves severe forms of antisocial behavior. Impacts of variables related specifically to children and youth with hearing impairments may be identified with less serious forms of maladaptive behaviors (eg. externalized behavioral problems).

Limitations

This study had a number of limitations. The study did not take into account the many variables that are associated with conduct disorders in children and adolescents. One of the most important, as we consider, is relation with parents and the general situation in family. This is related to a second limitation of the research. It has failed to learn the impact of specific characteristics of families of children with hearing impairments (primarily a way of communication and acceptance of a deaf child) that can be assumed to have effects on the development of conduct disorder. Research has failed to examine the relationship or other potentially relevant variables related to hearing loss (the time of initiation of rehabilitation, the development of sign language, the linguistic peculiarities and speech development). The study sample consisted of children who are educated in special forms of education, including isolation, lack of contact with normal hearing population, reduced educational expectations, and low assessment criteria and so on) or circumstances that may have affected the results of the research. Also, we were not able to attach the control related to the general characteristics of the environment (poor economic situation, transition, disrupted the system of values, the characteristics of the educational system) that could affect children and young people with hearing impairments and those without damage. Given that the environment variables are considered as possible determinants of the disturbance of conduct, we believe that their consideration in this research would be desirable.

Praxis Implications

The results of this study have implications relating to work with children and youth with hearing disorders and the prevention of potential developmental disorders and later psychopathology. Although the survey results did not indicate the prominent conduct disorder in children and adolescents with hearing impairment, we should not ignore the fact that certain indicators are more present than in children and young people without hearing loss. It would be important to check to what extent the presence of these indicators is a consequence of boarding lifestyle and isolated education that is available to a large number of children and youth with hearing impairments in Serbia.

Prevention programs that are expected to be able to have a positive impact on reducing the risk factors for occurrence of conduct disorders in children and adolescents with hearing impairments are related to psychosocial interventions. In schools for children and youth with hearing impairment it is advisable to conduct additional sports activities (especially for boys), and consider the possible positive impact of martial arts that would help control aggression and destructiveness. Art therapy and projective, non-directive non-verbal therapeutic techniques may be considered desirable for all children and youth with hearing impairments. In those who have stronger risk factors for occurrence of conduct disorders the additional psychotherapeutic intervention and family support is required. Prevention programs should be directed to the environment of children and youth with hearing impairments, particularly for reducing prejudice, given the research results (Dimoski, et al., 2013) demonstrated the presence of indifference and resistance to children and youth with impaired hearing. Preventive interventions for improving the academic achievement of children and young people with hearing impairment, according to research findings (e.g., Hawkins, Catalano, Kosterman, Abbott, & Hill, 1999) are in relation to a reduced risk of developing behavioral problems, including conduct disorders. Positive interventions in the education system in Serbia may have a potential very large positive impact because it would contribute to the development of inclusive trends that are still in their beginning. These changes would have a positive effect on strengthening the implicit self-esteem of children and youth with hearing impairments, reducing the risk of developing psychopathology, developmental age, including behavioral disorders.

Conclusion

This study did not find that children and young people with hearing impairments in Serbia have a higher presence of conduct disorders compared to children and youth with no damage. Findings suggest similar patterns of development of conduct disorders, regardless of hearing damage, since that established correlates of conduct disorders in hearing impaired children and young people this research detected with hearing population. Since conduct disorder involves serious manifestations of antisocial behavior, future research should examine the presence of developmental disorders that are characterized by less severe symptoms (externalizing disorder, behavior problems, socio-emotional problems) in children and adolescents with hearing impairment and determine any specificity in the occurrence related to hearing loss (method of communication during start-up and success of rehabilitation, acceptance of violence, experience with normal hearing peers, etc.). Also, future research should examine the presence and effects of risk factors of disturbance behaviors that have already been established in children and adolescents without impairments and their impact on children and young people with hearing impairment.

References

American Psychiatric Association. (2000). *Diagnostic and statistical manual of mental disorders.* 4th ed. American Psychiatric Association; Washington, DC: text revision.

Achenbach, T.M. (1996). Het cross-informant programma voor de CBCL/4-18, TRF & YSR [Computer software]. Burlington, VT: University of Vermont Department of Psychiatry (programmeurs: Arnold, J. en Jacobowitz, D.).

Achenbach, T. M., & Rescorla, L. A. (2001). *Manual for the ASEBA school-age forms and proles.* Burlington: University of Vermont,Research Center for Children, Youth & Families.

Bailly, D., Dechoulydelenclave, M.B., Lauwerier, L. (2003). Hearing impairment and psychopathological disorders in children and adolescents. Review of the recent literature. *Encephale.* 4 (1). 329-37.

Bardone, A. M., Moffitt, T. E., Caspi, A., Dickson, N., & Silva, P. A. (1996). Adult mental health and social outcomes of adolescent girls with depression and conduct disorder. *Development and Psychopathology, 8,* 811–829.

Barker, D.H., Quittner, A.L., Fink, N.E., Eisenberg, L.S., Tobey, E.A., Niparko, J.K. (2009). Predicting behavior problems in deaf and hearing children: The influences of language, attention, and partn-child communication. *Developmental Psychopathology.* 21(2).373-392.

Björkqvist, K., Lagerspetz, K.M.J., Kaukianen, A. (1992). Do girls manipulate and boys fight? Developmental trends in regard to direct and indirect aggression. *Aggressive Behav* 18:117–127.

Brooks-Gunn, J., Duncan, G. J., Klebanov, P. K.,& Sealand, N., (1993), Do neighborhoodsinfluence child and adolescent development?*American journal of sociology, 99,* 353-395.

Bursik, R. J., & Grasmick, H. G. (1993). *Neighborhoods and crime.* New York: Lexington Books.

Crick, N.R. (1995), Relational aggression: the role of intent attributions, feelings of distress, and provocation type. *Devalop Psychopathology.* 7. 313–322.

Crick, N.R., & Grotpeter, J.K. (1995). Relational aggression, gender, and socialpsychological adjustment. *Child Devalopmnt.* 66.710–722.

Cohen, P., Cohen, J., Kasen, S. Velez, C.N., Hartmark, C., Johnson, J., Rojas, M., Brook, J., Streuning, E.L. (1993). An epidemiological study of disorders in late childhood and adolescence, I: age and gender-specific prevalence. *J ournal of Child Psychologu and Psychiatry*. 34. 851–867.

Carr, A.(1999). *Handbook of Child and Adolescent Clinical Psychology: A Contecutal Approach.* London: Routledge.

Chase-Landsdale, P. L., & Gordon, R. A. (1996).Economic hardship and the development offive- and six-year-olds: Neighborhood andregional perspectives, *Child development, 67,* 3338-3367.

Dammeyer , J. (2009). Psychosocial Development in a Danish Population of Children With Cochlear Implants and Deaf and Hard-of-Hearing Children. *Journal of Deaf Studies and Deaf Education.* 15(1). 50-58.

Dimoski, S., Eminovic, F., Stojkovic, I., Stanimirovic, D., (2013). Contact with Persons with Hearing Impairments as a Correlate of Children's and Adults'Attitudes towards These Persons *Croatian Journal of Education.*15 (3). 611-628.

Dodge, K. A., & Pettit, G. S. (2003). A biopsychosocial model of the development of chronic conduct problems in adolescence. *Developmental Psychology, 39,* 349–371.

Duncan, G.J., & Brooks-Gunn, J. (1994). Economic Deprivation and Early Childhood Development. Child Development. 65 (2). 296–318.

Essau, C. A. (2003). Epidemiology and comorbidity. In C. A. Essau (Ed.), *Conduct and oppositional de!ant disorders: epidemiology, risk factors, and treatment.* Mahwah: Lawrence Erlbaum Associates, Inc.

Frick, P. J., Van Horn, J., Lahey, B. B., Christ, M. A. G., Loeber, R, Hart, E. A., et al. (1993). Oppositional defant disorder and conduct disorder: a meta-analytic review of factor analyses and cross-validation in a clinic sample. *Clinical Psychology Review, 13* (4). 319-340.

Frick, P. J., and Morris, A. S. (2004). Temperament and developmental pathways to conduct problems. *Journal of Clinical Child and Adolescent Psychology* 33: 54–68

Freeman, R. D., Malkin, S. F., & Hastings, J. O. (1975). Psychosocial problems of deaf children and their families: A comparative study. *American Annals of the Deaf. 120.* 275–304.

Friedrich, W.N., Urquiza, A.J., Beilke, R.L. (1984).Behavior Problems in Sexually Abused Young Children . *Journal of Pediatric Psychology*. 11(1).47-57.

Feehan, M., McGee, R., Raja, S.N., Williams, S.M. (1994). *DSM-III-R* disorders in New Zealand 18-year-olds. *Australian New Zeland Journal of Psychiatry.* 28.87–99.

Hawkins, D.J., Catalano, R.F., Kosterman, R., Abbot, R., & Hill, K.G. (1999). *Preventing adolescent health-risk behaviors by strengthening protection during childhood.* Archive of Pediatric and Adolescent Medicine.153(3). 226-34.

Hinshaw, S. P. (1992). Externalizing behavior problems and academic underachievement in childhood and adolescence: causal relationships and underlying mechanism. *Psychological Bulletin, 111* (1). 127-155.

Hinshaw, S. P., & Anderson, C. A. (1996). Conduct and oppositional defiant disorders. In E. J. Mash & R. A. Barkley (Eds.), *Child psychopathology* (pp. 113–149). New York: Guilford Press.

Hawkins, J. D., Smith, B. H., Hill, K. G., Kosterman, R. F. C., Catalano, F. C., & Abbott, R. D. (2003). Understanding and preventing crime and violence: Findings from the Seattle

Social Development Project. In T. P. Thornberry & M. D. Krohn (Eds.), *Taking stock of delinquency: An overview of findings from contemporary longitudinal studies* (pp. 255–312). New York: Kluwer Academic/Plenum Press.

Hausman, B. & Hammen, C. (1993). Parenting in homeless families: The double crisis. *American Journal of Orthopsychiatry. 63*(3), 358-369.

Hindley, P. A., Hill, P. D., McGuigan, S., & Kitson, N. (1994). Psychiatric disorder in deaf and hearing impaired children and young people: a prevalence study. *Journal of Child Psychology and Psychiatry. 35.* 917–934.

Hintermair, M. (2007). Prevalence of Socioemotional Problems in Deaf and Hard of Hearing Children in Germany. *American Annals of the Deaf. 152(3). 320-330.*

Ingoldsby, E. M., & Shaw, D. S. (2002). Neighborhood contextual factors and early-starting antisocial pathways. *Clinical Child and Family Psychology Review*. 5. 21–55.

Kerr, D.C.R., Lopez, N.L. Olson, S.L., Sameroff, A.J. (2004).Parental Discipline and Externalizing Behavior Problems in Early Childhood: The Roles of Moral Regulation and Child Gender. *Journal of Abnormal Child Psychology. 32(4). 369-383.*

Keenan, K., & Shaw, D. (1997). Developmental and social influences on young girls' early problem behavior. *Psychological Bulletin.* 121. 95-113.

Keenan, K., Loeber, R., Green, S. (1999). Conduct Disorder in Girls: A Review of the Literature. *Clinical Child and Family Psychology Review*. 2 (1). 3-19.

Kolvin, I., Fundudis, T., Spuy, H. I. J., Tweddle, E. G., & van der George, G. S. (1979). The hearing impaired child: Behavior and personality. In T. Fundudis, I. Kolvin, & R. F. Garside (Eds.), *Speech retarded and deaf children: Their psychological development.* (pp. 175–184). London: Academic Press.

Lahey, B.B, Schwab-Stone, M, Goodman, S.H, Waldman, I.D, Canino, G, Rathouz, P.J, Miller, T.L, Dennis, K.D, Bird, H, Jensen, P.S. (2000). Age and gender differences in oppositional behavior and conduct problems: a cross-sectional household study of middle childhood and adolescence. *Journal of Abnormal Psychology.* 109(3). 488-503.

Lahey, B.B., Miller, T.L., Gordon, R.A., Riley, A.W. (1999). Developmental epidemiology of the disruptive behavior disorders. In: *Handbook of the Disruptive Behavior Disorders,* Quay HC, Hogan A, eds. New York: Plenum, 23–48.

Loeber, R., & Schmaling, K. (1985). Empirical evidence for over tand covert patterns of antisocial conduct problems: a metaanalysis. *Journal of Abnormal Child Psychology. 13* (2). 379-390.

Loeber, R., and Wikstro m, P. H. (1993). Individual pathways to crime in different types of neighborhoods. In D. P. Farrington, R. J. Sampson, & P. H. Wikstrom (Eds.) *Integrating individual and ecological aspects of crime* (pp. 169–204). Stockholm, Sweden: National Council for Crime Prevention.

Loeber, R., & Keenan, K. (1994). Interaction between conduct disorder and its comorbid conditions: Effects of age and gender. *Clinical Psychology Review. 14.* 497–523.

Leventhal, T., and Brooks-Gunn, J. (2000). The neighborhoods they live in: The effects of neighborhood residence on child and adolescent outcomes. *Psychological Bulletin.* 126. 309–337.

Offord, D.R., Boyle, M.H., Szatmari, P., Rae-Grant, N.I., Links, P.S., Cadman, D.T., Byles, J.A., Crawford, J.W., Blum, H.M., Byrne, C. (1987). Ontario Child Health Study, II: six-month prevalence of disorder and rates of service utilization. *Archives of General Psychiatry.* 44. 832–836.

Offord, D. R., Alder, R., & Boyle, M. H. (1986). Prevalence and sociodemographic correlates of conduct disorder. *American Journal of Social Psychiatry. 6.* 272-278.

Parker, J. G., & Asher, S. R. (1987). Peer relations and later personal adjustment: Are low-accepted children at risk? *Psychological Bulletin. 102.* 357–389.

Patterson, G. R., & Yoerger, K. (1997). A developmental modelfor late-onset delinquency. In D. W. Osgood (Ed.) *Motivation and delinquency: Nebraska Symposium on Motivation* (pp. 119– 177). 44 Lincoln: University of Nebraska Press.

Peterson, D. R. (1961). Behavior problems of middle childhood. *Journal of Consulting Psychology*. 25(3). 205-209.

Prinstein, M.J., & La greca, A.M.(2004). Childhood Peer Rejection and Aggression as Predictors of Adolescent Girls' Externalizing and Health Risk Behaviors:A 6-Year Longitudinal Study. *Journal of Consulting and Clinical Psychology* . 72(1). 103-112.

Robins,L.N.(1966) *Deviant Children Grown-Up: A Sociological and Psychiatric Study of Sociopathic Personalities.* MD: Williams and Wilkins.

Robins, L.N., & Ratcliff, K.S. (1980). *The long-term outcome of truancy.* In L. Hersov & I. Berg (Eds.), *Out of school: Modern perspectives in truancy and school refusal* (pp. 65-83). New York: John Wiley.

Reiffe, C., Terwogt, M.M., Smit, C. (2003). Deaf Children on the Causes of Emotions. Educational Psychology: An International Journal of Experimental Educational Psychology. 23(2). 159-168.

Reiffe, C., & Terwogt, M.M. (2006). Anger communication in deaf children. *Cognition and Emotion.* 20.(8). 1261-1273.

Sampson, R. J.,& Groves,W. B. (1989). Community structure and crime: Testing social-disorganization theory. *American Journal of Sociology. 94*(4). 774–802.

Sinkkonen, J. (1994). Evaluation of mental health problems among Finnish hearing impaired children. *Psychiatrica Fennica. 25.* 52–65.

Stone, W L., & LaGreca, A. M. (1990). The social status of children with learning disabilities: A reexamination. *Journal of Learning Disabilities. 23.* 32-37

Stott, D. H. (1981). Behaviour disturbance and failure to learn: A study of cause and effect. *Educational Research. 23.*163-172.

Schlesinger, H.J., & Meadow, K. (1971). *Deafness and mental health: Developmental approach.* Berkeley, CA, itd: University of California Press.

Schonberg, M.A., & Shaw, D.S. (2007). Do the Predictors of Child Conduct Problems Vary by High- and Low-Levels of Socioeconomic and Neighborhood Risk? *Clinical Child and Family Psychology.* 10(2).101-36.

Sampson, R.J., Raudenbusch, S.W., Earls, F. (1997). Neighborhoods and violent crime: a multilevel study of collective efficacy. *Science.* 277. 918–924.

Stouthamer-Loeber, M., Drinkwater, M., & Loeber, R. (1999-2000). Family functioning profiles, early onset of offending, and disadvantaged neighborhoods. *International Journal of Child and Family Welfare*. 4. 247-256.

Tadić, N. (2010). *Psihijatrija detinjstva i mladosti.* Naučna knjiga. Beograd. (Psychiatry of childhood and adolescence. Scientific books. Belgrade).

Tremblay, R.E., Boulerice, B., Harden, P.W., McDuff, P., Perusse, D., Pihl, R.O., & Zoccolillo, M. (1996). Do children in Canada become more aggressive as they approach adolescence? In M. Cappe & I. Fellegi (Eds.), *Growing up in Canada.* Ottawa: Statistics Canada.

Meadow, K. P. (1980). *Deafness and child development.* Berkeley, CA: University of California Press.

Moffitt, T. E. (1993). Adolescence-limited and life-course-persistentantisocial behavior: A developmental taxonomy. *Psychological Review.* 100. 674–701.

Moffitt,T.E., Caspi, A., Dickson, N., Silva, P.A., Stanton, W. (1996). Childhood-onset versus adolescent-onset antisocial conduct problems in males: Natural history from ages 3 to 18 years.*Development and Psychopathology*. 8. 399-424.

Moffitt,T.E., Caspi, A., Rutter , M. and Silva, P.A. (2001) *Sex Differences in Antisocial Behaviour: Conduct Disorder, Delinquency, and Violence in the Dunedin Longitudinal Study*. Cambridge University Press.

Maes, B., & Grietens H. (2004). Parent-reported problem behavior among children with sensory disabilities attending elementary regular schools. *Journal of Developmental and Physical Disabilities.* 16. 361–375.

Meerum Terwogt, M., & Rieffe, C. (2004). Behavioural problems in deaf children: Theory of mind delay or communication failure?. *European Journal of Developmental Psychology.* 1. 231–240.

Masten, A. S., Coatsworth, J. D., Neemann, J., Gest, S. D., Tellegen, A., & Garmezy, N. (1995). The structure and coherence of competence from childhood through adolescence. *Child Development. 66.* 1635–1659.

Mitchell, T.V., & Quittner, A.L. (1996). Multimethod study of attention and behavior problems in hearing-impaired children. Journal of Clinical Child Psychology. 25(1). 83-96.

Mann, V. A., & Brady, S. (1988). Reading disability: The role of guage deficiencies. *Journal of 'Consulting and Clinical Psychology. 56.* 811-816.

Maguin, E., & Loeber, R. (1996). Academic performance and delinquency. *Crime and Justice: A Review of Research. 20.* 145–264.

Nagin, D., & Tremblay, R.E. (1999). Trajectories of boys' physical aggression, opposition, and hyperactivity on the path to physically violent and nonviolent juvenile delinquency. *Child Development.* 70(5).1181-96.

Quirin M., & Lane R. D. (2012). The construction of emotional experience requires the integration of implicit and explicit emotional process. *Behavioral and Brain Science.* 35. 159–160.

Žunić-Pavlović, V., Kovačević-Lepojvić, M., Pavlović, M. (2009). Procena socijalnog funkcionisanja učenika u školskoj sredini. *Nastava i vaspitanje.* 3(1). 399-420. (Assessment of social functioning of students in the school environment. *Teaching and Education.*)

Van Eldik, T. (1994). Behavior problems withdeaf Dutch boys. *American Annals of the Deaf. 139.* 394–399.

Van Eldik, T., Treffers, P. D. A., Veerman, J. W., & Verhulst, F. C. (2004). Mental health problems of Dutch children as indicated by parents' responses to the Child Behavior Checklist. *American Annals of the Deaf. 148.* 390–395.

Vostanis, P., Hayes, M., Di Feu, M., & Warren, J. (1997). Detection of behavioural and emotional problems in deaf children and adolescents: Comparison of two rating scales. *Child Care, Health, and Development, 23,* 233–246.

Van Gent T., Goedhart, A.W., Hindley, P.A., & Treffers, P.D.A.(2007). Prevalence and correlates of psychopathology in a sample of deaf adolescents. *Journal of Child Psychology and Psychiatry*. 48. 950–58.

Williams, S., & McGee, R. (1994). Reading attainment and juvenile delinquency. *Journal of Child Psychology and Psychiatry. 35*. 441–459.

Wikstrom, P.O. (1991). *Urban crime, criminals and victims*. New York: Springer-Verlag.

Wikstrom, P. O. (1998). Communities and crime. In M. Tonry (Ed.) *The handbook of crime and punishment* (pp. 269–301). NY: Oxford University Press.

Index

B

C

D

E

I

J

K

L

M

N

O

P

S